AIDS: Foundations for the Future

Social Aspects of AIDS

Series Editor: Peter Aggleton
Goldsmiths' College, University of London

AIDS: Foundations for the Future

Edited by
Peter Aggleton, Peter Davies and Graham Hart

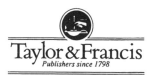
Taylor & Francis
Publishers since 1798

UK   Taylor & Francis Ltd, 4 John St., London WC1N 2ET
USA Taylor & Francis Inc., 1900 Frost Road, Suite 101, Bristol, PA 19007

First published 1994

A Catalogue Record for this book is available from the British Library

ISBN 0 7484 0227 6
ISBN 0 7484 0228 4 pbk

Library of Congress Cataloging-in-Publication Data are available on request

Series cover design by Barking Dog Art, additional artwork by Hybert ● Design & Type.

Typeset in 10/12pt Times
by Franklin Graphics, Southport

Printed in Great Britain by Burgess Science Press, Basingstoke on paper which has a specified pH value on final paper manufacture of not less than 7.5 and is therefore 'acid free'.

Contents

Contents

Preface

In July 1993, the seventh conference on Social Aspects of AIDS took place at South Bank University in London, bringing together researchers, health professionals and activists from many countries worldwide. Central amongst the issues examined was the extent to which adequate foundations for the future had been laid in community and voluntary sector responses, in health care policy and intervention, and in safer sex promotion. The meeting provided the opportunity to reflect on what has been achieved, barriers to effective work, and priorities for the future.

This book, like its predecessors in this series, contains key papers presented at the meeting. It serves both as a record of the conference, and as testimony to the collective effort currently underway to challenge the growing complacency which surrounds the epidemic. As editors, it has once again been a privilege to work closely with a professional and highly dedicated team, both in organizing the conference and in preparing the manuscript for publication. Our gratitude goes to Linda Alcaraz, Paul Broderick, Philip Gatter, Viv Gordon, Ford Hickson, Julian Hows, Peter Keogh, Vijay Kumari, David Reid, Jim Smith, Michael Stephens, Ian Warwick and Peter Weatherburn for pre-conference publicity and conference administration. Antoinette Dixon at South Bank University provided assistance well beyond the call of duty, and Helen Thomas liaised with authors and prepared the typescript with both skill and devotion.

Peter Aggleton
Peter Davies
Graham Hart

Chapter 1

An Anatomy of the HIV/AIDS Voluntary Sector in Britain

Jeffrey Weeks, Austin Taylor-Laybourn and Peter Aggleton

There appears to be widespread agreement on the importance of the voluntary sector in responding to the HIV/AIDS crisis, reflected in a variety of official policy statements, both national and international, and in a widespread popular recognition (Aggleton, Weeks and Taylor-Laybourn, 1993). This in turn reflects the role of the sector in defining the character of, and response to the health crisis from the early 1980s. In the earliest days of the epidemic it was an emergent alliance between voluntary groups (overwhelmingly drawn from the communities most affected) and public health officials that propelled the issue up the policy agenda in the mid-1980s (Berridge and Strong, 1991; Day and Klein, 1989). The voluntary sector pioneered a whole set of now taken for granted activities, from health education and prevention stategies, to practical support and direct services. As the National Audit Office (1991) noted:

> Service provision began in response to an emerging need identified by key hospitals and by a number of newly formed voluntary groups. These have continued at the forefront of providing care and support.
> (National Audit Office, 1991:10 para 1.6)

Voluntary agencies pioneered responses, and subsequently became vital partners to statutory bodies, nationally and locally, in the fight against the crisis. But this happy picture of collaboration between voluntary and statutory sectors conceals a number of shifts and changes over the period of the AIDS crisis, and a crucial ambiguity in the voluntary-statutory relationship. The early voluntary groupings, such as the Terrence Higgins Trust were formed because of the total absence of a coordinated national response, and the alliance with concerned public health officials was, as much as anything, a tactical alliance designed to put pressure on the government to recognize needs, and provide appropriate health education and services. The early voluntary provision was therefore

1

largely *faute de mieux*: voluntary services had to develop because, outside the hospitals and Genito-Urinary Medicine (GUM) clinics caring for people with HIV and AIDS, there was nothing else (Strong and Berridge, 1990). Indeed, a crucial element of the voluntary sector strategy was to campaign for the statutory sector to provide much needed services. The emergent voluntary sector was at first largely a substitute for absent services; a focus of pressure for better services; and a supplement to services which it was assumed could and should be provided through the community at large (that is, via the statutory sector).

Since the late 1980s there has been a dramatic increase in the size of the HIV/AIDS voluntary sector and of statutory provision, as the British government has responded to the dimensions of the crisis, and normalized HIV/AIDS-related service provision and policy following the 'war-time emergency' response of 1986 (Berridge and Strong, 1991). But the developing tendency of government policy has not in fact been to take over the voluntary provision but increasingly to encourage and support it as an *alternative* to statutory provision. In this the government response to the HIV/AIDS voluntary sector must be seen as part of wider policy developments (privatization, care in the community, contracting) to devolve welfare provision from the statutory sector to voluntary agencies and the informal sector. Thus the voluntary sector has assumed a critical importance not only because it has responded to perceived need at a time of crisis but because, for a series of factors, ranging from the fiscal crisis of welfarism to an ideology of privatization and self-help, the voluntary sector is seen as the best means of providing necessary services. But this, of course, puts a new burden on the voluntary sector as a whole, and on the great variety of organizations and groupings defining it, and in this respect the HIV/AIDS sector is no different from the voluntary sector as a whole.

The HIV/AIDS voluntary sector in Britain is thus important for two major reasons. In the first place it is important in its own right, as a prime focus for the response to a major new epidemic which had peculiar social, cultural and moral implications. In Britain at least, it largely affected unpopular and often execrated minority groups, gay men primarily, but also drug users and increasingly, minority ethnic communities in a climate where such groups were often, for quite other reasons, already targeted for a series of hostile, popular and sometimes governmental actions (Weeks, 1993). A study of the sector thus throws sharp light on the complexities of voluntary action in a climate marked by hostility and fear as an unprecedented epidemic threatened a rapid spread of debility, sickness and death in a wide population. But second, the role of the voluntary sector as a whole was undergoing radical changes as government sought to redefine the role of the welfare state in a situation of growing fiscal pressure and ideological redefinitions of the appropriate balance between individual needs, collective provision and state action. From this point of view, the HIV/AIDS voluntary sector offers a case study for investigating the shifting role of voluntary action as a whole.

This chapter is based on the first comprehensive study of the HIV/AIDS voluntary sector. Funded by the Economic and Social Research Council (grant

R 000233669), a research project entitled *Voluntary Sector Responses to HIV/ AIDS: Policies, Principles and Practices* has, since 1992, been conducting a two stage investigation into the work of the sector. In the first stage, the project team has conducted a questionnaire survey of nearly 550 voluntary agencies working around HIV and AIDS, with the aim of providing an anatomy of the sector. The second stage, currently in progress, will complement this survey with a series of case studies of specific voluntary agencies. This chapter offers a preliminary overall portrait of the HIV/AIDS voluntary sector as revealed in the survey. It is obviously limited by the absence of the in-depth qualitative material which will result from the second phase of the research, and therefore provides only a general picture of the sector. Nevertheless, we are able, on the basis of the initial survey, to highlight some key issues.

The first task of the research was to define the parameters of the project. The notion of the *voluntary sector* has, in the words of Perrie b (1991) long been 'clouded by conceptual confusion'. There is no agreed all-purpose definition of a voluntary agency either in statute or elsewhere, and there is no approximate equivalent definition in other English speaking countries. Definition is further complicated by constantly shifting boundaries between public, private and voluntary organizations. Billis (1989) has attempted a theory of the voluntary sector by defining three types of societal relationships: the personal, the associational and the bureaucratic. The personal broadly equates with private life (family, friends etc), the bureaucratic with the state and statutory agencies, and the associational with the voluntary. But in the HIV/AIDS sector, as in so many other parts of the voluntary world, the frontiers between these worlds are highly porous (see also Rochester 1992).

The first HIV/AIDS specific voluntary body in Britain, the Terrence Higgins Trust, was established by friends of Terrence Higgins, the first person to have 'officially' died of AIDS in Britain (Berridge, 1992), and throughout the history of AIDS organizations the link between personal friendships, personal needs, volunteering and organizational initiatives has been very close. Many other non-HIV/AIDS organizations no doubt have a similar genesis, but it is nevertheless a characteristic of many AIDS organizations that founding members had close personal ties, and certainly a common experience of illness, threat of illness, or the associated stigma. On the other hand, the natural history of many larger HIV/AIDS organizations has subsequently, in the view of a number of commentators, been characterized by a move towards greater managerialism and bureaucratization as the responsibilities of the organizations have increased and both the nature and funding of the agencies have changed. In this regard, there are many similarities with the wider range of voluntary bodies who have witnessed a parallel history.

Voluntary organizations have been defined by Fieldgrass (1992:1) as 'self-governing bodies of people who have joined together voluntarily to take action for the benefit of the community and have been established other than for personal gain.' This is a workable definition, but even here there are potential ambiguities. Many members of self-governing bodies, for example, are unpaid in that capacity, but may sit on a management committee by reason of their paid employment elsewhere, either in a voluntary or statutory agency. And paid employment and career possibilities in a voluntary agency are the norm rather than the exception; only a proportion are actually run by the volunteers themselves. The voluntary sector and volunteering are not the same, and must be sharply distinguished (Fieldgrass, 1992:14). Volunteering, as Hedley and Davis Smith (1992: ix) note, 'permeates all aspects of our daily life, and all activities' — including statutory provision. Contrariwise, while voluntary organizations often rely on volunteers, they are usually run by paid employees, and inevitably their patterns of organization often reflect wider organizational and managerial tendencies.

The ambiguities inherent in attempting to define the voluntary sector are underlined by the range of potential descriptions of 'self-governing bodies working for the benefit of the community': not-for-profit organizations, Non-governmental organizations (NGOs), Community-based organizations (CBOs), etc. All of these terms are used in relation to AIDS Service Organizations (ASOs), but they do not signify exactly the same things. NGOs, for example, have often been set up through governmental or inter-governmental initiatives; CBOs do not exhaust the range of ASOs. Furthermore, the HIV/AIDS sector in Britain has, like other needs-based areas, seen the emergence of a number of hybrid organizations. The Landmark centre in south-east London, for example, was established on the initiative of individuals working in the statutory sector, and its staff were managed and paid at first through the local health authority (Bebbington *et al.*, 1992). The National AIDS Helpline (NAH) was established following a telephone helpline initiative on BBC radio, is funded through the Health Education Authority (HEA), a statutory agency, and managed through Broadcasting Support Services, which in turn is closely related to the BBC, an independent national body governed by Royal Charter. CLASH (Central London Action on Street Health) was established explicitly as a partnership between statutory and voluntary agencies (Rhodes *et al.*, 1991). Yet the first of these organizations, Landmark, is normally seen as a voluntary body, the latter, CLASH, as statutory, with NAH as an ambiguous hybrid.

All of this suggests two essential elements we need to bear in mind in attempting to provide an anatomy of the HIV/AIDS voluntary sector. First, the HIV/AIDS sector is diverse. It ranges from small local groups, reliant on voluntary effort at all levels, to large national bodies, substantially or even wholly funded by statutory sources, from community-based self-help groups to quasi-statutory bodies. Second, the organizational history of the voluntary sector is constantly changing, implying a shifting relationship between the private, the voluntary and the statutory. This is reflected in the development of the individual organizations themselves, in their natural history, which is partly a result of internal developments, partly of the shifting relationship between government and statutory agencies and the voluntary organizations, and partly a result of the evolving role of the voluntary sector as a whole as an effect of developing social policy. These two elements will become clearer in the analysis that follows.

The diversity of the HIV/AIDS voluntary sector

The first task is to provide a brief overview of the size, distribution, and development of the HIV/AIDS voluntary effort, as revealed in the data from our survey. Perhaps the most important point to note here is the rapid growth of the HIV/AIDS voluntary sector, with specific organizations, such as the Terrence Higgins Trust, having an especially high recognition factor in public awareness of voluntary effort as a whole. This no doubt reflects the high profile of the epidemic itself over the past ten years, but also a recognition of the central role of the voluntary sector in responding to it.

Size of the Sector

For the first stage of our study, questionnaires were sent to 546 organizations that were identified as working in the broad field of HIV/AIDS. These organizations were selected from those listed in the National AIDS Manual (1992) and in the National AIDS Trust database, supplemented as appropriate by additional research and personal knowledge. This represented a sizeable voluntary sector in its own right (and is almost certainly an underestimate), and consisted of two broad divisions: HIV/AIDS specific organizations, especially established since the early 1980s as a direct response to the epidemic; and generalist organizations, which had a wider remit (for example, towards drug users or children), but which increasingly during the 1980s and early 1990s saw it as a vital part of their brief to address the challenges posed by HIV and AIDS. Completed questionnaires were received by the end of May 1993 from 224 organizations, a response rate of 41 per cent (subsequent late responses have not been included in the data that follow.)

The failure to respond in some cases can be explained by factors which are relevant to understanding the changing composition and role of the sector: some organizations had simply ceased to exist since the relevant databases had been compiled; others had changed their addresses, or lost their paid workers, or were over-reliant on extremely stretched volunteers. On the other hand, the survey also revealed the emergence of new groupings whose existence had not hitherto been widely noted. The sector, in other words, was still in rapid and dynamic evolution in the early 1990s.

Jeffrey Weeks, Austin Taylor-Laybourn and Peter Aggleton

Geographical Distribution

The HIV/AIDS voluntary effort is widely distributed throughout the United Kingdom, in a wide range of organizations. The early groupings that later became leading voluntary agencies in the HIV field were established in London, which was then, and continues to be the largest focus for HIV infection and AIDS cases (over 70 per cent of all United Kingdom reported cases of AIDS are in the two North London Regional Health Authorities). Not surprisingly, the largest grouping of voluntary agencies working around HIV and AIDS is concentrated in and around the capital and the four Regional Health Authorities centred on it. This distribution was broadly reflected in the response rate to the survey: 45.6 per cent of the organizations that responded are based in these four regions (a figure which is very close to the 47 per cent of the full sample of organizations identified as being based in the London area), while 33.5 per cent are based in just two of the RHAs, North East Thames and North West Thames.

It follows that half the remaining agencies are based outside the London health regions, with significant concentrations in Scotland (7.6 per cent), the South Western Region (7.4 per cent), the West Midlands (7.0 per cent) and Yorkshire (5.8 per cent). It is noteworthy that some of the lowest concentrations of organizations working around HIV and AIDS were the Trent (2.2 per cent), Northern (1.3 per cent) and Northern Ireland (0.9 per cent) Regions.

Two points are important here. First, the largest concentrations of organizations are, on the whole, in the regions with the largest conurbations, and therefore containing populations likely to be most at risk. In fact, by coincidence, the percentage of the UK cumulative total of reported AIDS cases between January 1982 and July 1993 in the Northern RHA is 1.5, remarkably close to the overall percentage of responding voluntary agencies. Second, however, the distribution may also reflect the fact that outside the larger cities and regions, there tends to be a concentration of voluntary activity in fewer multi-function HIV/AIDS specific agencies, while by comparison, London has a much wider range of specialist HIV and generalist organizations responding to particular needs, and also the largest organizations, including the Terrence Higgins Trust and the London Lighthouse.

The majority of the organizations that responded (58 per cent) defined themselves as HIV/AIDS specific, but that still leaves a sizeable proportion that are generalist in orientation. However, some 42 per cent of these generalist organizations specified their main work as being drugs related, while another 28.4 per cent defined their main concern as being about advice and counselling on sexual issues (this grouping consisted almost exclusively of lesbian and gay switchboards, support and counselling groupings such as Friend, or bisexual groups). In other words, over half of the generalist organizations came from fields that were closely related to the main focuses of the epidemic, leaving only some 32 per cent of the generalist sample (22 per cent of the sample overall) to represent other areas of concern.

Evolution of the sector

It is possible to hypothesize a series of phases in the history of the HIV/AIDS voluntary sector. There have been several attempts to categorize the various phases of the response to HIV/AIDS as a whole (see Weeks, 1991; Berridge and Strong, 1991), with a general agreement that 1986 saw a qualitative shift in the governmental response, with a period of emergency mobilization followed by a period of crisis management, normalization or stabilization of public policy. Obviously, the history of the voluntary response is related to this, but also has to be related to wider social policy shifts. For convenience we can tentatively identify three phases (the dating is even more tentative, and disguises a great deal of variation geographically, in terms of constituency and services provided, and considerable overlap of the phases).

Constructing a voluntary response: 1983–86

This was a period defined by a mobilization of concern, a definition of need over a whole range of potential services, a massive reliance on voluntary effort, and limited public funding.

Creating a service culture: 1987–90

This period was characterized by a considerable expansion of the AIDS specific sector and services, and a broadening of HIV/AIDS concerns and activities into the generalist sector; a substantial increase of funding levels, with Section 64 funding and AIDS Support Grants; and the development of collaborative initiatives across the voluntary and statutory sectors; the legitimization and survival of (most of) the HIV/AIDS voluntary sector, but also the emergence of acute organizational and managerial crises as the sector adjusted to new demands.

Jeffrey Weeks, Austin Taylor-Laybourn and Peter Aggleton

Adapting to a contracting culture: 1991–94

The main feature of this period was the emergence of a contracting culture. By this is meant the adaptation by the voluntary sector to the UK government's new policy, enshrined in the National Health Service reforms and the development of care in the community policies, which involved the ending of a grant regime and its replacement by the negotiation of contracts between *purchasing* statutory agencies and *providing* service organizations, often, but not exclusively, voluntary. At the time of writing, the evidence of the impact of this shift is still sketchy, but its impact is potentially great, with voluntary agencies increasingly competing with statutory and private sector organizations to provide services. These developments promise to have a profound effect on the HIV/AIDS sector, both in terms of threats to AIDS specific funding, and on the managerial and organizational priorities of voluntary agencies. At the same time, needs continue to increase, and to be redefined (for example, in terms of changing constituencies at risk, recognition of equal opportunity issues, etc).

Some of these issues will be discussed later in this chapter, but at this stage our aim is to show how these phases relate to the evolution of the sector as a whole. In fact, some 37 per cent of the organizations which responded to the survey were founded in the first phase of the crisis, but only half of these were HIV/AIDS specific. Of those groups founded after 1986, however, over 80 per cent were HIV/AIDS specific. In the survey as a whole, only four HIV/AIDS specific organizations claimed to be more than 10 years old, compared to 37 generalist organizations. This, of course, simply reflects the recent nature of the epidemic, and the well established nature of many of the more generalist agencies.

The natural histories of HIV/AIDS voluntary organizations

At each phase of their development, HIV/AIDS voluntary agencies have been forced to adapt to survive. Some have collapsed under the strains (for example, Frontliners; see Moreland and Legg, 1992). Others have undergone crises of management or funding (see National AIDS Trust 1992). Others have adjusted as best they can. Our aim in this section is to indicate some of the main forces at work in shaping these developments.

In terms of service provision, HIV/AIDS voluntary agencies are generally seen as having a number of advantages over other bodies (Fieldgrass, 1992: 15; see also Bebbington *et al.*, 1992: 29ff), for example, greater flexibility of structure and approach; a sense of vision; the experience of being close to the 'customer'; experience of being users; a patchwork of different kinds of organizations, from national to local, from advocacy to direct service provision; the opportunity to experiment and innovate; the commitment to being flexible and opportunistic (in the sense of taking advantage of opportunities); a greater sensitivity to equal opportunity issues; and a commitment to openness of information, making information simple, and sharing it. But clearly, the ability to fulfil such promises depends on a host of factors, and two factors in particular stand out. First, there are ambiguities relating to the voluntary sector in general. Thus Kramer notes that a voluntary agency is:

> a curious hybrid of an organisation, mixing three, seemingly incompatible elements: a service bureaucracy, a voluntary membership association, and informal personal relationships — all in one structure. To complicate matters, it also maintains two parallel lines of authority, between board and staff, and between professionals and volunteers, in its governance and management.
>
> (Kramer, 1990:13)

All these characteristics are displayed in the history of HIV/AIDS organizations, but have been compounded by the specific circumstances of the epidemic including stigma, uncertain public and governmental response, illness and death, and 'burn-out'.

Second, the stage of development of the individual organization is important in determining its responsiveness to the above concerns. The HIV/AIDS specific groupings had their origin in a sense of personal commitment and concern, often directly involving people affected by HIV. They frequently emerged as self-help and advocacy organizations, and established services (information lines, 'buddying', mutual support, training, care, etc.) to plug gaps and satisfy directly felt or perceived need. But the skills and abilities needed for this stage of growth (personal involvement, dedication, charismatic founders) were not necessarily the qualities needed to take the organization on to the later stages of development. Moreland and Legg commented on the rise and demise of Frontliners in the following terms:

> Due to its rapid growth Frontliners found itself in the position of trying to evolve from 'birth' to 'maturity' by rushing through the learning stage of 'childhood' and by missing out 'adolescence' altogether.
>
> (Moreland and Legg, 1992: 15, Appendix A)

This suggests a natural progression through stages which is unnessarily deterministic, and there is plentiful evidence in the voluntary sector that refutes such a picture. Nevertheless, it is undoubtedly the case that many organizations have experienced serious strains as they have 'matured', and adapted to new circumstances.

Changing priorities

The earliest HIV/AIDS specific organizations were either advocacy or campaigning groups, though with significant nascent service functions (particularly the provision of advice), of which the Terrence Higgins Trust is the classic example, or self-help groups of and for people with HIV or AIDS, such as Body Positive, which also developed related service-type activities (newsletters, drop-in centres, social events and so on). As the sector has developed, however, the organizations, and the services offered, have become increasingly complex. The survey asked organizations to indicate their aims and objectives. These ranged from providing practical and emotional support, the provision of health education information and raising general awareness about HIV/AIDS, to providing training, financial support and affecting policy changes. The vast majority of respondents indicated their commitment to more than one of these categories, though with significant emphases reflecting the particular history of the sector. Thus, for instance, 51 per cent indicated that they aimed to provide practical and emotional support, 37 per cent the provision and dissemination of HIV/AIDS related health education, and 10 per cent helping to 'empower people affected by HIV/AIDS'. On the other hand, only 3 per cent indicated that their aim was to 'affect policy changes relating to HIV/AIDS'. This in part reflects the formal structure of a large percentage of organizations as charitable trusts, which limits overt political action.

These aims and objectives must be balanced, however, by the actual services provided. Our data indicate the overwhelming commitment (by 77 per cent of respondents) to providing health education information, just over half providing counselling and external training, almost half providing helplines and befriending services, a third providing alternative therapies, financial support and legal advice, and over 28 per cent offering drop-in facilities. These figures indicate the wide range of activities and services provided by the HIV/AIDS related voluntary sector, and the difficulty of fitting organizations into neat categories.

Just as the services provided are diverse, so are the target groups, reflecting a sense of the general threat posed by the epidemic. Layzell and McCarthy (1992: 203) have noted: 'AIDS has presented social policy makers with an unprecedented challenge: to provide comprehensive care sensitively and flexibly to an increasingly diverse client group.' HIV/AIDS services have developed in response to the recognition and articulation of needs, and have changed as needs have changed, grown, and spread to diverse client groups. The development of HIV/AIDS services has been widely seen as a model for services in health-related and care approaches generally (National Audit Office, 1991, Department of Health 1992). But it has also led to a growing recognition of the different needs of different populations at risk, posing questions about the sensitivity of services to these needs, and questions of equal access to provision (see Bhatt,

1992). This in turn has stimulated the emergence of new voluntary groups, attending to the needs of women, black people, gay men, etc.

The data from our survey does suggest, however, that there are problems in these developments. Indeed, a number of respondents objected to the invitation to indicate the highest priority for targeted service delivery. As one respondent put it: 'We deal with priorities for activities/services and needs; *not* client groups; we are opposed to discrimination and we provide specific services for *all* people with HIV disease.' In fact, 44 per cent suggested that their 'highest priority' was serving the 'general HIV constituency', with 30 per cent also emphasizing the priority given to 'gay/bisexual men' and 27 per cent injecting drug users; 23 per cent gave highest priority to women, 20 per cent to children and young people, 9 per cent to people from minority ethnic communities, and 5 per cent to people with haemophilia. The figures are not exclusive, as a number of respondents indicated more than one top priority.

It is worth noting, for comparison, the relative modes of transmission of actual AIDS cases between 1982–93: 74 per cent were infected through sexual intercourse between men, 7.3 per cent were cases of women through various sources, 4.8 per cent were amongst injecting drug users, and 4.8 per cent amongst people infected through contaminated blood products (for example, people with haemophilia). Explicit data on the number of people from minority ethnic communities with HIV or AIDS, cutting across these categories, is not easily available, but it is clear from anonymized data that ethnic minorities are disproportionately represented among recent evidence for heterosexual transmission of HIV. The evidence of our survey would tend to suggest that the existing distribution of voluntary agencies broadly reflects the main areas of risk and the key areas where services are needed. There is not sufficient evidence from our data, however, to indicate whether services are being provided in proportion to the real and anticipated need. Evidence from elsewhere suggests that the development of generalist services prevents the targeting of resources on areas of greatest need, especially among gay men (King, Rooney and Scott 1992). This is part of a more general debate which is addressed below.

Organization and management

The HIV/AIDS-related organizations have had diverse origins, and differing trajectories within a common history both of reactions to HIV and social policy developments. But all the organizations have had to face sharp challenges to their organization, structure and management, and a changing role for volunteers (see National AIDS Trust, 1992, National Audit Office, 1991). Bebbington *et al.*, (1992: 196) suggest that, despite such changes, 'the underlying purpose is still the essential ingredient'. This is undoubtedly true, but it is equally true that organizations have often changed dramatically in the process. In particular, commentators have seen a widespread pattern of professionalization, bureaucratization and a growing managerialism, which in turn have given rise to internal conflict and cultural shifts, a changing relationship between management, paid employees and volunteers, and a potentially changing relationship between organizations and the communities and client groups to which they relate.

Perhaps surprisingly, the survey itself did not clearly confirm this picture. When asked to indicate the main challenges faced by the organization a) in the early years, and b) in the last year, specific management issues were given a very low priority. Only 3 per cent of the voluntary agencies named such issues as a major challenge for the early years, and 6 per cent for the past year. Similarly, broader questions of organizational structuring did not feature significantly: 20.5 per cent suggested structure had been a major challenge in the early years (perhaps not surprisingly, given the difficulties of setting up an organization), but only 11 per cent highlighted this as a major problem in the past year. The major problem in both periods was establishing a secure financial base: 47 per cent in the early years, compared to 41 per cent for the later period.

This lack of emphasis on specific management issues perhaps reflects the fact that the majority of those who completed the questionnaires were senior managers or coordinators of the organizations concerned, and therefore by nature of their role were likely to see such issues in a different light from paid workers and volunteers. Evidence from a workshop held as part of the project (*Maintaining Momentum, 1993*) confirms that questions of management and structure were indeed important to voluntary agencies, and this is a topic that will be more intensively studied in the case studies of Phase 2 of the research project. However, three overlapping management issues may be identified: relations between the formal management committee or equivalent and paid managers and workforce; the relationship between senior managers and workers; and the relationship between the organization as a whole and volunteers.

A very high proportion of the voluntary agencies define themselves as charities (66.5 per cent), while only 10 per cent defined themselves as 'informal groupings' (generally local support groups). 28.5 per cent of the total were registered as limited companies. The vast majority therefore were bound by a formal constitution and status, which specified the responsibilities of the managing group. Echoing this distribution, 62 per cent were governed by management committees, and only 19 per cent through membership meetings. There seems to be a strong correlation between size of a group (defined for this purpose in terms of numbers of paid workers) and formal structure — the smaller the group, the more likely it is to be governed by meetings of members; the larger, the more likely that it is governed formally by management committees.

Size of the agency is an important factor in relationship to other key factors. Overall, amongst the responding organizations, 28 per cent had no paid workers (and hence have been defined as small); 26 per cent had between 1 and 3 paid workers (small-medium), 29 per cent had between 4 and 10 paid workers (medium-large), and 17 per cent had over 10 (large), with 9 per cent having more than 15 paid workers. However, when these figures are broken down into HIV/ AIDS specific and generalist organizations, it becomes clear that on the whole the former are smaller than the latter. For example, 37 per cent of the HIV/ AIDS specific organizations fall into the small-medium grouping, compared with 14 per cent of the generalist. By contrast, 20 per cent of the generalist organisations fall into the large groups category, compared with 8 per cent of HIV/AIDS specific organizations. This probably reflects both the more recent histories of most HIV/AIDS specific voluntary agencies, and the more directed nature of their work. For instance, for most generalist organizations (the exceptions being the drug agencies and the gay and lesbian helplines), HIV/ AIDS activity is only a relatively small part of the work.

Size of an organization is also obviously linked to its geographical location and 'reach'. As might be expected, HIV/AIDS-specific organizations based in the Thames Health Regions, the epicentre of the epidemic, tend to have larger paid workforces: 24 per cent of Thames based organizations have more than 10 paid workers, compared to 11 per cent nationwide. Similarly, if we break the data down by a national/local 'reach', we find that 47 per cent of local HIV/ AIDS specific groups had one or no paid workers, compared to 15 per cent of national groups (usually, though not invariably, based in London), with a similar workforce.

What the data does suggest is that, with a few notable exceptions, management problems that tended to occur are in organizations which cannot in any way be defined as large, and problems are therefore more likely to be about the crucial transition from informal to formal structures, and from none or just a few paid workers to a relatively small number, than about the problems of managing very large organizations.

In categorizing the size of an organization we have used the criterion of number of paid workers. This is, of course, only part of the picture: it does not take into account the use of volunteers. The early HIV/AIDS-specific organizations began as volunteer bodies. Subsequently, many of the key functions were either taken over by paid workers or organizations were established with fully paid workforces, largely with statutory funding support. However, the majority of organizations (91 per cent of our sample had more than 10 volunteers) continue to rely on substantial volunteer labour (see Sharma *et al.*, 1992), though this is not clearly related to an organization's size or income. For example, there seems to be no significant relationship between the number of volunteers involved in an organization and its income. Indeed, 52 per cent of organizations with less than ten volunteers had incomes of over £100 000 per annum. Only eight organizations had more than 100 volunteers, though five of these had more than 500. The critical measure of volunteer involvement appears to be function: the groups, regardless of size, with the highest number of volunteers are those involved in direct services: befriending, help with practical matters at home, counselling and training. The changing role of volunteering will need further investigation in the next phase of the project.

Funding

Funding issues have been crucial to the development of the HIV/AIDS voluntary sector. Before what Street (1993) calls the '1986 watershed', grants to the HIV/AIDS voluntary sector were few and far between. In 1985–86, direct funding from the Department of Health to the HIV/AIDS voluntary sector totalled £35 000. Subsequently there was a substantial increase. Between 1985–6 and 1992, central government granted some £8.9 million through the Section 64 provisions of the Health Services and Public Health Act (1968) to voluntary organizations in the HIV field. During the same period over £500 million was made available through the HIV budget head and the AIDS Support Grant (ASG) to health authorities for 'prevention, treatment and care', some of which was redistributed to the voluntary sector for services and by way of grants (Department of Health, 1992). In the sample of HIV/AIDS voluntary organizations surveyed by The Volunteer Centre 79 per cent of income came from statutory sources (Sharma *et al.*, 1992). But these global figures conceal real funding difficulties. As the National Audit Office report (1991: 3) noted, 'the funding mechanisms in England for the voluntary sector are unclear.' Funding could come from a variety of sources, each with a different mechanism for assessment and different criteria for giving grants, demanding multiple applications. Funding levels varied from year to year, and the continuation of funds was always uncertain. Even within the North West Thames Regional Health Authority, with a very high proportion of the national AIDS cases, only some £150 000 from the ASG was distributed to voluntary organizations in 1990–91. Funding levels, moreover, were not always shaped by actual need but by political decisions, and more closely related to the government's fiscal problems.

The announcement in early 1993 by Virginia Bottomley, the Secretary of State for Health, of the proposed capping of the amount obtainable under Section 64 funding to a maximum of £150 000 per annum has severe financial implications for the larger HIV/AIDS organizations, namely the Terrence Higgins Trust and the London Lighthouse, while the phasing out of ear-marked HIV/AIDS funding from April 1994 threatens the stability of many smaller organizations dependent on winning contracts from the statutory sector. This is at a time when the cases of AIDS continue a steady growth, and the HIV figures suggest a much larger epidemic in the next five to ten years.

The data from our survey (which covered the financial year 1991–92) indicates in fact two key points. The first is that income from voluntary sources is substantial. If we look at the HIV/AIDS-specific organizations alone, we can see that 16 per cent of organizations received more than half their income from voluntary initiatives, while 54 per cent received up to half their income from such sources. But the corollary of this is that at the same time there is a heavy reliance on statutory sources. Some 24 per cent of agencies received over half their income from district health authorities, 12 per cent over half from regional health authorities, and 16 per cent the majority of their income from local authorities. Any threat to statutory sources of income is, therefore, likely to make the stability of the sector as a whole extremely precarious.

The other crucial point to make is that the HIV/AIDS voluntary sector is not particularly well-financed, with, it has been estimated, less than 0.2 per cent of charitable donations in the UK going to AIDS-related charities. Nearly half (48 per cent) of the HIV/AIDS-specific organizations in our survey had incomes of less than £50 000 in 1991–2; 28 per cent had incomes of less than £10 000, and some 8 per cent of the total had incomes of less than £1000 per annum. Within these global figures there were, however, interesting regional differences. In the London/Thames regions only 18 per cent of organizations had less than £10 000 a year; but this rose to 40 per cent nation-wide.

These data suggest that the funding basis of the sector remains broadly insecure, and the qualitative data in the survey indicates a growing concern with funding-related questions, particularly relations with statutory bodies and the problems of adjusting to a contracting regime. One-fifth of the voluntary agencies surveyed reported that 'just surviving' was their primary concern for 1993–4, while half stated that their major problem was simply 'maintaining momentum'. Clearly, questions concerned with financial stability were central to such anxieties. This brings us to the heart of the policy questions facing the HIV/AIDS voluntary sector — issues of policy.

Policy issues

As we have argued above, the policy context operates across two axes: the evolving attitude towards HIV/AIDS, both in general terms and in relation to particular communities and individuals at risk; and the development of public policy in general. The first is specific to HIV/AIDS organizations and activities, but in turn, policy towards these is to a large extent shaped by government attitudes, the political and economic context, and shifts in social policy towards health, the role of the non-statutory sector, funding levels and so on. This dual context is crucial to the understanding of the policy issues that seem currently to be coming to the fore. At least three related issues recur in the literature and are reflected in the data from our survey. We simply note them here; a more detailed discussion will be found in subsequent publications.

The impact of the contracting culture

Throughout the 1990s, suggests Kramer (1990: 8), 'voluntary agencies are likely to be viewed by Government more as a substitute service provider or public agent; a preferred alternative, rather than, as in the Wolfenden (1978) Report a decade ago, as a supplement to statutory provision'.

Contracts, Kramer argues (1990: 8), 'are distinguished by tighter, more explicit and rigorous criteria for funding'. They establish a 'quasi-market' relationship between purchaser of services and providers (which will include the voluntary sector).

These changes raise a number of key issues: the evolution of 'care in the community' policies and the new role assigned in these to voluntary agencies; the relations between voluntary and statutory bodies; the impact of contracting on levels of funding and organizational culture in the voluntary organizations. The changes are likely to have major effects on the working of the HIV/AIDS sector, offering opportunities for some organizations, but also major challenges. Bebbington *et al.* (1992: 205) are sceptical of the positive effects: 'what has become clear is that despite the rhetoric, these provisions of the Act [1990 NHS and Community Care] may present HIV/AIDS organizations with as many problems as opportunities'. Fears have been expressed, for example, that contracts will not be offered to agencies that are too political; or, a related possibility, statutory agencies may simply offload responsibility in politically or culturally delicate areas, such as around race and minority ethnic communities (Bhatt, 1992). At the same time, the task of negotiating contracts with a myriad of statutory bodies can be daunting, problems which are compounded when an organization has a national reach.

Key questions therefore include: to what extent have relations with the statutory sector changed; is there more collaboration, joint planning of services; what sorts of tensions arise; is the purchaser-provider division working; to what extent has tendering and contracting forced changes in the operation of the organization; has it narrowed the focus of the group, forced the toning down of advocacy or campaigning; has it had benefits for the organization; how is it going to affect the sector as a whole? Our survey does not provide answers to these questions, but there are indications (reflected in Craig and Hopper, 1990; *Maintaining Momentum, 1993*) that they increasingly preoccupy the sector.

Mainstreaming

Questions of contracts in turn raise issues concerning the special role of the sector, and whether HIV/AIDS services could best be delivered through their mainstreaming into more generalist organizations, both statutory and voluntary. As Brazier has put it:

> Initially, HIV was considered a 'problem' to be dealt with by specialist HIV/AIDS agencies. However, as such groups have become increasingly stretched and the number of people affected by HIV has

continued to grow, more generalist agencies have become aware of the need to integrate HIV related issues into their work.

(FIAC, nd.: 6)

The mainstreaming of HIV work has obvious advantages, particularly in the stress it puts on HIV/AIDS as a problem that the whole community must face, regardless of the groups particularly affected. But at the same time, it has dangers, especially if the result is to marginalize or endanger the specialist HIV services that have developed.

For the generalist agencies it raises a number of key issues: training, staff and managerial awareness, the development of relevant outside links, funding for new services, questions of confidentiality, monitoring and evaluation of new services, etc. For the specialist agencies it raises more delicate questions: has it marginalized or threatened the specialist services, and in what ways; will it affect levels of funding; is it possible to forge links with generalist agencies; has it heightened awareness of HIV-related issues, or led to them being absorbed into wider questions of health and care? These questions in turn point to the issue of how best to target services to those most in need.

Targeting

The implications of government reforms of the NHS and the development of a contract culture has been to emphasize the need to target resources on those with most need. At the same time, activists, especially from the gay community, have expressed alarm that generalized HIV education and funding has tended to marginalize the needs of those still most at risk (see King, Rooney and Scott 1992; King, 1993). Targeting has two apparently related but different implications: one largely concerned with effective resource allocation and value for money; the other fuelled by a feeling that real needs are being neglected, in a climate that is still shaped by a reluctance to target resources to unpopular or marginalized groups. It is necessary, therefore, to explore the implications of targeting: what are its effects on the HIV/AIDS specific and generalist voluntary agencies; is there evidence that statutory bodies are reluctant to support organizations targeting unpopular groups; does targeting stigmatize vulnerable groups; how do voluntary organizations counter this?

The data we currently have do not provide answers to these questions; they provide, however, the research agenda which guides the research of the second case-study phase of our research. What can be said is that the HIV/AIDS voluntary sector, after a period of rapid growth, is now facing major challenges as the policy context and the related funding regimes change significantly. The history of the sector so far suggests that some organizations will be unable to survive the challenges, others will survive, although, not without further organizational shifts. Beyond that is a further question, which lurks in the brief discussion above on mainstreaming: whether the sector as a whole, in its current shape, size and diversity, has a long term future as a distinctive part of the voluntary sector. The history so far suggests that it should; the challenge facing the HIV/AIDS sector is to ensure that it does.

References

AGGLETON, P., WEEKS, J., TAYLOR-LAYBOURN, A. (1993) 'Voluntary responses to HIV and AIDS: A framework for analysis', in AGGLETON, P., DAVIES, P. and HART, G. (Eds) *AIDS: Facing the Second Decade*, London: Falmer Press.

BEBBINGTON, A. C., FELDMAN, R., GATTER, P., and WARREN, P. (1992) *Evaluation of the Landmark: Final Report*, Canterbury: University of Kent, PSSRU Discussion Paper 901/2.

BERRIDGE, V. (1992) 'The early years of AIDS in the United Kingdom 1981–6', in RANGER, T. and SLACK, P. (Eds), *Epidemics and Ideas*, Cambridge: Cambridge University Press.

BERRIDGE, V., and STRONG, P. (1991) 'AIDS policies in the UK: A study in contemporary behaviour', *Twentieth Century British History*, **2**, 2, pp. 150–74.

BHATT, C. (1992) 'Empowerment and understanding: HIV prevention work with black and minority ethnic communities', in EVANS, B., SANDBERG, S. and WATSON, S. (Eds), *Working Where the Risks Are: Issues in HIV Prevention*, London: Health Education Authority.

BILLIS, D. (1989) *A Theory of the Voluntary Sector: Implications for Policy and Practice*, London: London School of Economics, Centre for Voluntary Organizations, Working Paper 5.

FIAC (nd) *Into the Mainstream, Developing Generalist Services in the Light of HIV and AIDS*, BRAZIER, A. (Ed.) London: Federation of Independent Advice Centres.

CRAIG, M. and HOPPER, C. (1990) *HIV/AIDS Services in the Contract Culture*, London: London Voluntary Services Council.

DAY, P. and KLEIN, R. (1989) 'Interpreting the unexpected: The case of AIDS policy making in Britain', *Journal of Public Policy*, **9**, 3, pp. 337–53.

Department of Health (1992) *HIV Infection: The Working Interface between Voluntary Organisations and Social Services Departments, 1991–2*, Social Services Inspectorate/HIV Unit, London: Department of Health.

FIELDGRASS, J. (1992) *Partnership in Health Promotion: Collaboration Between the Statutory and Voluntary Sectors*, London: Health Education Authority/National Council of Voluntary Organisations.

HEDLEY, J. and DAVIS SMITH, J. (Eds) (1992), *Volunteering and Society: Principles and Practice*, London: NCVO Publications, Bedford Square Press.

KRAMER, R. (1990) *Voluntary Organisations in the Welfare State: On the Threshold of the '90s*, London: London School of Economics, Centre for Voluntary Organisations, Working Paper 8.

KING, E. (1993) *Safety in Numbers: Safer Sex and Gay Men*, London: Cassell.

KING, E., ROONEY, M., SCOTT, P. (1992) *HIV Prevention for Gay Men: A Survey of Initiatives in the UK*, London: North West Thames Regional Health Authority.

LAYZELL, S. and McCARTHY, M. (1992) 'Community-based health services for people with HIV/AIDS: a review from a health service perspective', *AIDS Care*, **4**,2, pp. 203–15.

Maintaining Momentum (1993) Report of a Workshop held on 28 September 1993, organized by the Voluntary Reponses to HIV/AIDS Project Team, London: Institute of Education, University of London, Health and Education Research Unit.

MORELAND L. and LEGG, S. (1992) *Managing and Funding AIDS Organisations: Experience from the Closure of Frontliners*, London: Compass Partnership for the Department of Health.

National AIDS Manual (1992) *Directory*, London: NAM Publications.

National AIDS Trust (1992) *Report on the Management Development Programme, 1990–1991*, London: National AIDS Trust.

National Audit Office (1991) *HIV and AIDS Related Health Services: Report by the Comptroller and Auditor General*, London: HMSO.

PERRIE B (1991) *What is a Voluntary Organisation? Defining the Voluntary and Non-Profit Sectors*, London: NCVO.

RHODES, T., HOLLAND, J., HARTNOLL, R. (1991) *Hard to Reach, or Out of Reach: An Evaluation of an Innovative Model of HIV Outreach Health Education*, London: The Tufnell Press.

ROCHESTER, C. (1992) 'Community organisations and voluntary action', in HEDLEY, J. and DAVIS-SMITH, J. (Eds) *Volunteering and Society: Principles and Practice*, London: NCVO Publications, Bedford Square Press.

STREET, J. (1993) 'A fall in interest? British AIDS policy, 1986–1990', in BERRIDGE, V. and STRONG, P. (Eds), *AIDS and Contemporary History*, Cambridge: Cambridge University Press.

SHARMA, S., DIXON, S., DAVIS SMITH, J. (1992) *Volunteering in HIV and AIDS Organisations: A Report of a Survey*, Voluntary Action Research Paper No 6, Berkhamsted: The Volunteer Centre.

STRONG, P. and BERRIDGE, V. (1990) 'No one knew anything: some issues in British AIDS policy', in AGGLETON, P., HART, G. and DAVIES, P. (Eds), *AIDS: Individual, Cultural and Policy Dimensions*, London: Falmer Press.

WEEKS, J. (1991) *Against Nature: Essays on History, Sexuality and Identity*, London: Rivers Oram Press.

WEEKS, J. (1993) 'AIDS and the regulation of sexuality', in BERRIDGE, V. and STRONG, P. (Eds), *AIDS and Contemporary History*, Cambridge: Cambridge University Press.

Wolfenden, J. (1978) *The Future of Voluntary Organisations*, London: Croom Helm.

Chapter 2

The Changing Context of Health Care in the UK: Implications for HIV/AIDS

Neil Small

There are numerous, and often competing, histories of AIDS (Berridge and Strong, 1993). These histories include the medical and the scientific, the political and public histories of the epidemic, and those private histories of people affected by HIV-related illness. My concern in this chapter is with the recent history of the public policy response to HIV/AIDS. Public policy exists on two fundamental levels — at the level of *assertion* and at the level of *action*. There is a framework of legislation and regulation within which public policy in relation to HIV/AIDS exists, but within that framework there is room for manoeuvre. How this is interpreted can have far reaching effects on the overall experience of service providers, service users and on the public perception of the urgency, even the reality, of the epidemic.

The political and economic imperatives that underpin public policy are influenced by scientific, medical and epidemiological debates about HIV/AIDS. They are further influenced by public opinion and pressure group activity. We have seen, in the history of responses to HIV/AIDS in the UK, these different forces impacting upon the overall picture to varying degrees. The result has been that many commentators have identified distinct periods in which different influences are in relative ascendancy. Strong and Berridge (1990) identified a first period in which the emergency gradually became visible, followed by a second phase of major, if selective, intervention by central government. Weeks (1989) approaches the early history rather differently in that he uses it to demonstrate that state policy in relation to HIV/AIDS reflected an era in which a 'new right' government, engaged in a crusade against what it defined as the (im)moral excesses of the 1960s and 1970s, engaged with the problem as a moral panic, and initiated meaningful action only when it appeared clear that the heterosexual population was at risk. Government sought to incorporate responses within a dominant professional medico-social paradigm which devalued the already considerable contribution of self-help groups.

In the USA Fee and Kreiger (1993) have identified two phases in the construction of the history of AIDS and then described the different implications for health and social policy of each of these. This schema has resonances in recent developments in the UK. AIDS was initially seen as an epidemic disease, a *gay plague*. The resulting sense of emergency had an ambiguous impact — it generated an allocation of funds, allowed some opening of dialogue on sex and saw the emergence of some gay groups who were able to assert a place in the discourse of response and treatment. But it also allowed for draconian methods of prevention and social exclusion. In the USA, constructing AIDS as a sudden and time limited emergency allowed the government to justify taking money from other funds in order to respond to AIDS, while still seeking to contain overall health expenditure.

Second, AIDS was then normalized as a chronic disease, similar in many ways to cancer. This phase allowed health professionals to re-assert their expertise. Specialist AIDS units were set up in an institutionalization of the disease that shut some doors to gay groups and prevented new groups, for example, African Americans and women entering the policy arena. Scarcity of funds was emphasized, and a considerable interest displayed in accurate estimates of need and the calculation of the costs of care. There were four further features of this phase. First, a concern with pursuing new treatments, although activists were still having to fight for speedier protocols and better availability of current treatments. Second, there was an increase in the centrality of arguments in favour of HIV antibody testing, reflecting a belief that knowledge of one's status had some positive implications for treatment. Third, there was a decrease in the generally perceived sense of risk from casual transmission and fourth, there was an increase in concerns about health care workers who were antibody positive, for example surgeons and dentists, having contact with patients.

Fee and Kreiger suggest a third phase may develop, wherein AIDS is constructed as a slow-moving, long-lasting pandemic, a chronic infectious ailment manifested through myriad but specific HIV-related diseases. This change recognizes both the communicable aspects of the disease and its chronic nature. Its communicable features require that sexuality and drug use must be better understood as integral to long term strategic provision with risk behaviour understood in terms of cultural meanings and social context. Mass education programmes targeted at multiple communities must be devised and disseminated. Its chronic aspects require secure finding and the development of services in collaboration with local communities.

Identifying varying phases in the response to AIDS implies some sort of linear history. But the picture is more complex. The layered nature of differing discourses that surround HIV/AIDS and the absence of a dominant framework by which we incorporate HIV/AIDS into the public sphere means that any phase in the history of AIDS is only tentatively achieved — the history is contested, it is fluid. Phase models of history imply some metamorphosis from one stage to another — a caterpillar becomes a moth. But a better analogy is a beehive — at its centre is the virus and the people touched by it. But buzzing around, making noise, attracting attention, are many different views — the one closest to you at the time attracts your attention. But different perceptions come and go, replaced by others. Some of these views link to public perceptions of science, to medicine, while others involve stigma, constructed as popularist scares.

In the recent histories of HIV and AIDS in the UK, one can see a most pronounced fluidity. With this are many of the features described by Fee and Kreiger but without the assumptions of 'progression'. We have seen an important debate about likely future incidence of HIV/AIDS. On the one hand it suggested that there is not as big a problem as had been predicted, particularly for the heterosexual population. Others see the pattern of the epidemic in Britain as indicative of a developing and substantial problem. The same data are used to support both positions. For example, a report prepared by Nick Day of the Institute of Public Health in Cambridge was used on 21 May 1993 by the *Independent* to underline the reality of heterosexual AIDS in the UK. A few days earlier *The Sunday Times* (9 May 1993) used the same figures (of between 20 000 and 30 000 people infected with HIV in the UK) to argue that the epidemic was of lesser severity than even the most conservative official estimates of six or seven years ago.

A second major debate has been around the efficacy of the anti-viral drug AZT when prescribed to delay the progress of symptomatic disease in HIV seropositive people. *The Lancet* (3 April 1993: 889–90) reported results of the Concorde trial. AZT does not significantly delay the onset of AIDS or AIDS-related diseases and does not increase the chances of survival of HIV-infected people. While AZT would still be prescribed for people with AIDS the focus of treatment for the wider group would shift even more towards combinations of drugs. While the Concorde results appeared to shock the Stock Exchange, the reaction elsewhere was rather one of re-orientation towards the longer term search for effective treatments.

A third feature of the recent public debate about HIV/AIDS has been a series of stories in the press about health care workers with AIDS. These stories were invariably accompanied by reassurances from employers that risks to patients were very slight but that telephone helplines would be made available to respond to patient anxiety. The government reacted to these stories, and to the generalized atmosphere of scare that accompanied them, by changing guidelines so that health authorities had a duty to inform patients who may have been at risk from doctors and medical workers who were HIV seropositive (Recom-mendations of the Expert Advisory Group on AIDS, 1993).

The debate about rates of increase and the likely pattern of spread within the heterosexual population, the sense of disappointment — if not surprise — at the setbacks in treatment and the scares around contagion are all resonant of features of the history of AIDS as described by Fee and Kreiger. We have seen how they argue that the way AIDS is understood, both as a medical condition and a social phenomenon, has implications for the development and implemen-tation of policy. I will go on to look at the most significant areas for the development of health and social care in terms of the legislative framework but here will consider those changes in policy implementation, and particularly the allocation of government money, that can be linked directly to the changing picture of AIDS that dominates at any one time.

Recent policy changes

In May 1993, Health Secretary Virginia Bottomley announced a change of strategy on AIDS. The Grant that had been paid to the Terrence Higgins Trust (THT) and to the London Lighthouse would be cut from £450 000 to £150 000. This was because 'the feared HIV epidemic among heterosexuals had not materialised' (Bottomley, 1993). Resources would be targeted on the 'high risk groups — homosexuals and drug abusers'. The cut was also justified as consistent with AIDS' new status as a health problem that had to be seen alongside other illnesses, 'We do not need to give it the kind of pump-priming priority as when it was a new and strange disease.' The Secretary of State also argued that the government's health education campaigns had succeeded, comparing British experience with that in Paris, where there were 1.5 times as many AIDS cases as in the whole of the UK.

Responding to the Secretary of State's announcement, Les Rudd, Director of the National AIDS Trust, interpreted the changes in funding as being indicative of an attack on a soft target by a Minister responding to Treasury calls for spending cuts. He also pointed to a lack of logic in saying 'a policy has been successful therefore we will now curtail it'. John Nicholson, Director of the George House Trust, in a letter to the *Guardian* (6 May 1993) argued that it would be progress indeed if AIDS were to be treated purely as a health issue alongside other health issues. But to achieve this barriers of prejudice would have to be removed, poverty and deprivation attacked and positive health promotion and care developed for stigmatized groups.

In its first reactions to the arrival of AIDS as an issue of concern, the British government did allocate funds, but much of this allocation was seen as short-term and was achieved by redirecting funds from other sources. At the same time although some support was given to self help groups, this was done in an environment of heightened prejudice — media scares, discrimination, violence, the exclusion of gay groups from Ministerial press conferences, seizure of health education literature at the ports, along with punitive legislation, including Section 28 and Clause 25 (Small, 1988). All this is consistent with Fee and Kreiger's first phase, as is the shift to set up alternative avenues of response that are incorporated in the mainstream both ideologically and institutionally. Schramm-Evans (1990) chronicles how the Department of Health and Social Security pressured the management of the National AIDS Helpline to 'broaden its counselling base' — in effect to stop relying on counsellors who had come from the Helpline from the THT or from Gay Switchboard, even though they were the most knowledgeable about HIV, AIDS and allied issues.

A governmental wish to shift from supporting approaches that emphasize empowerment, a characteristic of the self help and much of the voluntary sector response to HIV/AIDS, into a more contained and controlled orthodox professional response is accompanied by an absence of recognition that lessons learned by specialist organizations like the THT and the London Lighthouse are transferrable into the wider development of health education, health care and care in the community (Small, 1993a and 1993b). Progressive reductions in funding to the THT and London Lighthouse cannot simply be understood as evidence of attempts to cut costs. The sums involved are very small. Since 1985–6 central government has provided, through Section 64 of the Health Services and Public Health Act 1968, funding of £8.9 million directly to voluntary organizations in the HIV field. In addition both central and local authorities have, at the behest of central government, made grants available to those same or similar voluntary organizations. In the former case this has been through a specifically identified HIV budget, and in the latter, through the AIDS Support grant payable to Local Authority Social Services Departments. It is estimated that £510 million had been made available from central government to the NHS and Local Authorities for prevention, treatment, care and support costs. A further £199 million had been allocated for the financial year 1992–3 which included £15.3 for the AIDS Support Grant (Department of Health 1992c). Expenditure for 1993–4 was announced as £250 million (*Sunday Times*, 9th May 1993).

The approach towards HIV/AIDS illustrates Fee and Kreigers' first two phases. It veers between treating HIV/AIDS as a dangerous interloper and its sufferers as stigmatized outsiders, and one that seeks to incorporate responses within unchallenging professional paradigms. Such a policy is carried out according to the changing profiles and prejudices that characterize the public position of HIV/AIDS. But they are also carried out within a context of a more fundamental, legislatively structured, reorganization of the health service and of community care. I will continue with an examination of the three crucial legislative initiatives *Working for Patients, The Health of the Nation* and *Caring for People*. In so doing I will consider how far the government was moving towards the third of Fee and Kreigers' phases where a policy emerges that takes cognizance of the need for a long term prevention strategy and for sensitive and flexible care in a variety of settings.

Working for patients

The 1989 White Paper *Working for Patients* (Department of Health, 1989a) set in place the subsequent division of the NHS into purchaser and provider units and the establishment of fundholding General Practitioners. It was very much a continuation of a shift towards an enhanced managerialism that had begun in the major reorganization of health services in 1974 (see Ham, 1985: 26) and had been boosted by the appointment of general managers after the 1983 *Griffiths Report* (DHSS, 1983). The introduction of market principles into the day to day practice of the NHS was a significant innovation, destined to have a long term impact on both the way health care was organized and the way it was experienced by service users. By 1993, in England, one person in four had a fundholder for a GP. The number of NHS Trusts has increased very rapidly; the first wave was of 57 units, the second of 9, and the third 128. By mid-1993 most hospital provision was located in Trusts.

As long ago as 1975, Alford (1975) identified three sets of structural interests in health care politics. First, *dominant*, doctors as professional monopolists; second, *challenging*, managers and planners as corporate ratio-nalisers; and third *repressed*, patient and consumer groups. One can see recent NHS reforms as facilitating 'attempts by "corporate rationalisers" to respond to public and professional concern about the under-funding of the NHS by the promise of greater output without significantly greater input' (Williams *et al.*, 1993: 64). Using Alford's categorization, the challengers now have a structure and ideology — general management, internal markets, efficiency savings, performance indicators, resource management — that allows them to vie for the position of dominant interest (c.f. Harrison *et al.*, 1990: 161). At the very least, there is now a contested dominance. We are still awaiting the eventual outcome.

Ferlie and Pettigrew (1990) report a study carried out in what was then Paddington and North Kensington District Health Authority (DHA). Their concern was to see how a DHA responded to a major new health care issue — the arrival of AIDS in the 1980s. Their analysis is pre- *Working for Patients* but includes the period in which general management was introduced in this DHA–1985. They conclude that 'the overall trend is for the transfer of ownership of the issue from clinical to managerial arenas' (Ferlie and Petti-grew, 1990: 199). Certainly within this district, and in central London more generally, one can attribute the development of a consciousness of the problem of AIDS to pressure from two directions. First, from Alford's repressed interests — the consumers and potential consumers of services. Second, from clinicians. There were letters to *The Times*, approaches to Department of Health advisory groups and the early publication of the findings of research teams based in central London (see Pinching *et al.*, 1983; Cheingsong-Popov *et al.*, 1984). In contrast, the ascendent structural interest, managers, may have been introduced in part to help the NHS move more quickly, one of the aims identified in the Griffiths Report, but that movement emphasized the pursuit of value for money and efficiency and not the development of progressive strategic service change.

Working for Patients sought to extend patient choice and affirm that the patients' needs were paramount. Both choice and the elevation of patients' needs were to be achieved via the establishment of a market in health care whereby health care would be bought on behalf of patients by either health authorities or fundholding general practitioners. Provider units (increasingly NHS Trusts) would negotiate contracts and seek to develop services consistent with their own assessment of need and expertise, but essentially they would provide the services that the purchasers wished to buy. This proxy empowerment of service users raises three as yet unanswered questions. What means will purchasers devise to ascertain the needs and wants of the populations for which they are responsible? If we assume that wants will outstrip the means to meet them then how will decisions about rationing be made? How can the health service move from a concern with the costs of inputs to measures of how health interventions relate to outcomes, both for individuals and populations?

It is not surprising that these questions have not been answered, as they remain problems for health care systems everywhere. But they have a special relevance for the development of services for HIV and AIDS. An early anxiety about *Working for Patients* was that GPs would turn away potential patients who were HIV-positive or had AIDS on the grounds that they would involve high levels of expenditure for the practice. Second, provider units would not prioritize expenditure on services for a stigmatized minority. In reality there remains some anxiety about access to good primary care, along with concern about the willingness of purchasers to refer patients to the facility of their choice. A patient may want to seek treatment in a hospital or other facility, such as a hospice, with which the purchasing authority does not have a contractual relationship. Extra-contractual referrals are possible, but it is becoming clear that purchasers are developing a reluctance to agree to all requests for this sort of service. Patients may want to seek treatment outside the area in which they live for a variety of reasons. Anonymity and confidentiality are of tremendous importance for some. So too is the pursuit of what is seen as a specific expertise. We have therefore a clash of goals — patient choice versus cost control — that is illustrative of the core problem in the market principle of determining the allocation of health care.

It is not a problem that can be reconciled by looking at outcomes because the question of cost remains. Health economists, Eastwood and Maynard (1990) suggest that one has to consider the benefit of medical interventions in terms of the quality and the length of life after treatment alongside cost. In an article entitled 'Treating AIDS: Is it ethical to be efficient?' they conclude,

> If the objective of the NHS is to maximise improvements in health, then resources should be allocated on the basis of general benefit . . . and least cost. The consequence of this rule . . . is that patients with illnesses such as end stage renal failure and AIDS might be left untreated.
>
> (Eastwood and Maynard, 1990: 246)

With a problematic relationship to all but a committed cohort of doctors, and with managers intent on cost cutting the third interest group in health care politics becomes of crucial importance — the consumer. Here we can see, for example, some effective representation from the Haemophilia Society and from the groups campaigning for people given infected blood by the NHS who were not haemophiliacs (Small, 1993b: 81). There are also excellent examples of the many groups including THT, Body Positive and Positively Women which have grown up in response to the epidemic. But as I have argued above, these have had an uneasy relationship with health policy makers and have been under attack. Their voice needs to be heard in a dialogue about service development. If it is not, then *Working for Patients* will not be working for these patients.

The health of the nation

As well as the development of managerialism and market principles, recent years have seen an extension, in legislation and Department of Health policy guidance, of health promotion and disease prevention as central aims of the health service. *Promoting Better Health* (Secretaries of State for Social Services *et al.*, 1987) the new contract for GPs (Department of Health, 1990) and *The Health of the Nation* (Department of Health, 1992a) all represent important steps in reclaiming a role for the state and the health service in the promotion of health.

The Health of the Nation identifies a health strategy for England based on the identification of key areas where intervention in terms of both health promotion and changes in procedures and practice can reduce premature morbidity and mortality. The areas chosen to concentrate resources were: cancers; coronary heart disease and strokes; mental illness; accidents; and HIV/AIDS and sexual health. This final category was decided upon somewhat belatedly — it was not included in the Green Paper discussion document that preceded the White Paper but when it was included it came with the clear statement that 'HIV infection represents perhaps the greatest new public health challenge this century' (Department of Health, 1992b).

The *Health of the Nation* is essentially a series of targets. In relation to HIV/AIDS and sexual health two such targets illustrate the general approach. First, a reduction in the incidence of gonorrhoea in men and women aged between 15 and 64 by at least 20 per cent by 1995, from 61 cases per 100 000 (the 1990 figure) to no more than 49. Second, a reduction in the percentage of injecting drug users who share equipment from an estimated 20 per cent (1990) to 10 per cent by 1997 and to 5 per cent by the year 2000.

The proposed five-part programme is to facilitate the achievement of these targets. Prevention is to be promoted via public awareness campaigns; community based initiatives; education in schools and colleges, and improved prevention and treatment services for injecting drug users. There was to be monitoring, surveillance and research to improve the knowledge of the epidemiology, transmission and natural history of HIV. Treatment, care and support including adequate education and support for professionals and volunteers is integral to the programme as is a recognition of the importance of social, legal and ethical issues. There is a need to foster a climate of understanding and compassion, to safeguard confidentiality and to discourage discrimination. Finally, the importance of international co-operation is included in the programme. This is an impressive list. Indeed *Health of the Nation* goes further. It recognizes that the pursuit of these and other targets requires the active involvement of other sectors of society. Health is not just the responsibility of the health service. Much is made of the need to foster interdepartmental links and to develop 'alliances for health' involving NHS bodies, local government, the voluntary sector and business.

So far so good. But there are problems. First, is setting targets the best way to achieve change of the sort required? Here expert opinion is divided (Williams *et al.*, 1991). The alternative is to emphasize means and not be preoccupied with ends. David Player, Secretary of the Public Health Alliance, has argued that, 'Targets can be useful in themselves by injecting a touch of accountability and discipline in those who announce them.' (*Independent*, 5 June 1991). Second, there is a concern with the targets chosen. They might be a public relations device of little meaning in terms of health performance. Either they concern areas difficult to measure, like statistical reduction in childhood accidents in a health district, or they might simply reflect the continuation of existing trends — targets will be reached because that is the way the incidence curve is moving. It is also possible that having these targets means that the government does not have to grasp the implications of the World Health Organization's 38 'Health for All by the Year 2000' targets. These are much more politically challenging putting, as they do, the reduction in inequalities top of the target list.

Other reservations might relate to the idea of alliances. These could be construed as means for health bodies to exercise some sort of hegemony over a wide range of environmental concerns. Inter-agency groups often become the means for the most powerful to exercise control over other bodies not previously within their orbit. Local Government might well resent such attempts at takeover and point to the value of their own initiatives in projects like *Healthy Cities*. Finally, the government sees the post- *Working for Patients* NHS as providing the necessary mechanisms for achieving *The Health of the Nation* targets. Contracts can insist on achievements in these areas, the market and a combination of the carrot and the stick making things move in the desired direction.

The aims of *The Health of the Nation* in relation to HIV/AIDS and sexual health are to be welcomed. Achieving the targets would require a valuable shift. The incidence of gonorrhoea does fluctuate but, give the time span involved, the government can not rely on cyclical processes to achieve its target. Likewise the reduction in needle sharing is significant. One hopes that emerging alliances will include users and carers.

Caring for People

A wish to reform care in the community has been an agenda item for many years. It is something that has bridged the political divide in that there has been a shared wish to shift from institutional care to care in the community where at all possible. Part of the imperative to effect some change comes from the changing demographic profile of the population, with the realization that the cohort of the very elderly will increase markedly. In part the shift has come from a realization of the shortcomings of institutional care and the desire of many to stay in the community. *Caring for People* (Dept. of Health, 1989b) sought to effect care in the community via the encouragement of a mixed economy of care. At the heart of this change was a shift of role for local authorities. They would be transformed from providers of services to enabling authorities setting up and supporting these mixed economies (Wistow *et al.*, 1992) .

Caring for People has four key features. Primary responsibility for managing community care is to be given to local authorities. Acute care and care of the terminally ill will remain within the remit of the health service. There will be a division between the purchasing and providing functions of local government. Care management will be introduced, as will better quality assurance. In addition there is to be, on the part of statutory authorities, a responsibility to promote the mixed economy of care including taking steps to stimulate the setting up of not-for-profit agencies and to stimulate the development of new voluntary sector activity.

Caring for People offers an opportunity for developing and supporting imaginative care for people with HIV and AIDS. Voluntary sector activity, not-for-profit organizations, offer the opportunity for responsive services linked closely to local need and the specifics of user choice. But taking the opportunity presented is not straightforward. The new arrangements for community care have been framed with the interests of other client groups in mind — specifically the elderly. People with AIDS are mentioned only fleetingly in the Act. Further, the new system relies on the development of voluntary sector activity via the purchasing activity of statutory services. But, as Bebbington *et al.* (1992) have argued, statutory authorities have to take some responsibility for fostering, supporting and resourcing not-for-profit organizations. It is not enough simply to say money is available. The experience of the USA is that statutory bodies have to recognize that developing services takes a lot of time, that it may not be possible to generate many service providers and that a number of different patterns of support must be considered (Kramer and Grossman, 1987).

Even if not-for-profit organizations are established there are still continuing problems that need to be addressed. First is the need to communicate accurately what service is being offered and to whom. Getting enough appropriate referrals is crucial — one problem is that an innaccurate image of the service to be offered develops and serves, in a self-perpetuating way, to limit the usefulness of the agency. An example might be a perception in potential referrers that an agency offers a service only to gay men. This may not be consistent with the self image of the agency but will impact upon its potential to attract a wide range of referrals. Second is the way that an ongoing relationship between purchaser and provider develops in terms of scrutiny of the latter by the former. There is a possibility that the very variety and flexibility that are the strengths of the not-for-profit sector will be compromised by interventionist purchasers defining the details of service delivery.

In the longer term three main questions arise. First, how will new agencies deal with the uncertainty caused by having to plan around short term contracts? Second, will all propensity to innovation be located in this sector, leaving established statutory services devoid of new ventures and new thinking? Third, will cost rather than quality dominate long term contracting strategies?

Like *The Health of the Nation, Caring for People* has the capacity to lead to improvements in services for people with HIV and AIDS. It could facilitate the development of voluntary sector activity that would replicate and build on some of the best examples of response so far evident. It could encourage collaboration between health and social care at the statutory level and inform commissioning and contracting that would mean services could be developed according to need, rather than according to the dominant institutional structures and service attitudes. But it could also perpetuate insecurity for voluntary groups and oppressive intervention by purchasers.

It is at this point that an assessment of *Caring for People* and *Health of the Nation* has to be made in the light of the market approach of *Working for Patients*. The various concerns considered above come together in a realization that their effectiveness is predicated on a market model. It is this that underpins them and it is to this that I return.

Conclusion

The impact of the changes to the NHS, introduced since 1990, have still to be assessed. A recent conference noted a reluctance on the Department of Health's part to evaluate their effectiveness. At that conference there was a recognition that the reforms could 'degenerate into the commercial free-for-all that many fear. Or they could take on a momentum of their own and improve the process of planning and delivery' (Nick Bosanquet, quoted in May, 1993)

There was also a strong sense that two paradoxes lay at the heart of the reforms. First they were designed to make the NHS more efficient and yet expenditure on general and senior management had increased dramatically — by 109 per cent between 1990 and 1992 — according to Jeremy Lee-Potter, Chair of the British Medical Association (*The Guardian*, 29 June, 1993). Second, they were ostensibly designed to introduce freedom from central control and yet, as John Butler has put it, it is 'a market strictly controlled from the desk of the Secretary of State' (May, 1993). It should also be noted that debates about appropriate levels of funding and about equity and inequalities in health have been sidelined in the debates emerging from the structural changes in the NHS.

If we return to the model of phases in constructing a history of AIDS presented by Fee and Krieger, referred to earlier, we can see that in the UK, HIV/AIDS has not entered that period in which it can be responded to as both chronic and communicable disease, even though there are elements in *Caring for People* and *The Health of the Nation* that directly address these aspects of HIV/AIDS. Rather, responses to HIV/AIDS oscillate between the stigmatizing, the institutionalizing and the possibility for synthesizing. This last possibility, which would see alliances for health developing between professional and self-help groups, between service providers and service users, is undermined by two fundamental forces. First, a market orientation that serves to elevate managerial interest above professional or patient interests. Second is an environment in which the reforms are implemented. This includes ideological pressure and public opinion which perpetuates the stigmatization of AIDS.

I have argued here that the public environment within which policy in relation to HIV and AIDS is enacted is volatile. The legislation described has a strategic trajectory but, although elements in it are to be welcomed, the general direction of change should give rise to concern for those people seeking to respond effectively to the health and social care needs generated by HIV and AIDS.

References

ALFORD, R. (1975) *Health Care Politics*, Chicago, IL: University of Chicago Press.

BEBBINGTON, A.C., FELDMAN, R., GATTER, P. and WARREN, P. (1992) *Evaluation of the Landmark*, Personal Social Services Research Unit, Discussion Paper 901/2, Canterbury: University of Kent.

BERRIDGE, V. and STRONG, P. (1993) (Eds) *AIDS and Contemporary History*, Cambridge: Cambridge University Press.

BOTTOMLEY, V. (1993) The World at One, BBC Radio 4, 3 May.

CHEINGSONG-POPOV, R., WEISS, R.A., DALGLEISH, A., TEDDER, R.S., JEFFRIES, D.J., SHANSON, D.C., FERNS, R.B., BRIGGS, E.M., WELLER, I.V.D., MITTON, S., ADLER, M.W., FARTHING, C., LAWRENCE, A.G., GAZZARD, B.G., WEBER, J., HARRIS, J.R.W., PINCHING, A.J., CRASKE, J., BARBARA, J.A.J. (1984) 'Prevalence of Antibody to Human T-Lymphotropic Virus Type III in AIDS and AIDS risk patients in Britain', *The Lancet* 1 Sept, pp. 477–83.

DEPARTMENT OF HEALTH (1989a) *Working for Patients*, Cm 555, London: HMSO.

DEPARTMENT OF HEALTH (1989b) *Caring for People*, Cm 849, London: HMSO.

DEPARTMENT OF HEALTH (1990) *General Practice in the NHS: A New Contract*, London: HMSO.

DEPARTMENT OF HEALTH (1992a) *The Health of the Nation*, London: HMSO.

DEPARTMENT OF HEALTH (1992b) *The Health of the Nation Key Area Handbook: 7*, London: HMSO.

DEPARTMENT OF HEALTH (1992c) *The HIV Infection. The Working Interface between Voluntary Organisations and Social Service Departments*, London: Social Services Inspectorate, The AIDS Unit.

DEPARTMENT OF HEALTH AND SOCIAL SECURITY (1983) *NHS Management Inquiry (Griffiths Report)*, London: HMSO.

EASTWOOD, A., MAYNARD, A. (1990) 'Treating AIDS. Is it ethical to be efficient?' in BALDWIN, S., GODFREY, C. and PROPPER, C. (Eds) *Quality of Life: Perspectives and Policies*, London: Routledge and Kegan Paul.

EXPERT ADVISORY GROUP ON AIDS (1993) 'AIDS-HIV Infected Health Care Workers', London: Department of Health.

FEE, E. and KREIGER, N. (1993) 'Thinking and rethinking AIDS: Implications for health policy', *International Journal of Health Services*, **23**, 2, pp. 323–46.

FERLIE, E. and PETTIGREW, A. (1990) 'Coping with change in the NHS: A frontline district's response to AIDS', *Journal of Social Policy*, **19**, 2, pp. 191–220.

HAM, C. (1985) *Health Policy in Britain* (2nd Ed.) London: Macmillan.

HARRISON, S., HUNTER, D. and POLLITT, C. (1990) *The Dynamic of British Health Policy*, London: Unwin Hyman.

KRAMER, R.M., and GROSSMAN, B. (1987) 'Contracting for social services: Process management and resource dependencies', *Social Service Review*, **61**, pp. 32–55.

MAY, A. (1993) 'Atheists, agnostics and believers', *Health Service Journal*, 15 April, p. 11.

PINCHING, A.J., JEFFRIES, D.J., DONAGHY, M., MUNDAY, P.E., MCMANUS, T.J., MOSHTAEL, O., PARKIN, J.M., HARRIS, J.R.W. (1983) 'Studies of cellular immunity in male homosexual in London', *The Lancet*, **ii**, 16 July, pp. 126–29.

SCHRAMM-EVANS, Z. (1990) 'Responses to AIDS, 1986–1987', in AGGLETON, P., HART, G. and DAVIES, P. (Eds) *AIDS:Individual, Cultural and Policy Dimensions*, London: Falmer Press.

SECRETARIES OF STATE FOR SOCIAL SERVICES, WALES, NORTHERN IRELAND AND SCOTLAND (1987) *Promoting Better Health: The Government's Programme for Improving Primary Care*, London: HMSO, CMND 249.

SMALL, N. (1988) 'AIDS and social policy', *Critical Social Policy*, **21**, pp. 9–29.

SMALL, N. (1993a) 'HIV/AIDS: Lessons for policy and practice', in CLARK, D. (Ed.) *Death and Dying: Future Issues in Policy and Practice*, Buckingham: Open University Press.

SMALL, N. (1993b) *AIDS: The Challenge. Understanding, Education and Care*, Aldershot: Avebury.

STRONG, P. and BERRIDGE, V. (1990) 'No one knew anything: some issues in British AIDS policy', in AGGLETON, P., HART, G. and DAVIES, P. (Eds) *AIDS: Individual, Cultural and Policy Dimensions*, London: Falmer Press.

WEEKS, J. (1989) 'AIDS: the intellectual agenda', in AGGLETON, P., HART, G. and DAVIES, P. (Eds) *AIDS: Social Representations, Social Practices*, Lewes: Falmer Press.

WILLIAMS, S.J., CALNAN, M. and CANT, S. (1991) 'Health promotion and disease prevention in the 1990s', *Medical Sociology News*, **16**, 3, pp. 20–9.

WILLIAMS, S.J., CALNAN, M., CANT, S.L. and COYLE, J. (1993) 'All change in the NHS? Implications of the NHS reforms for primary care prevention', *Sociology of Health and Illness*, **15**, 1, pp. 43–67.

WISTOW, G., KNAPP, M., HARDY, B., ALLEN, C. (1992) 'From providing to enabling: local authorities and the mixed economy of social care', *Public Administration*, **70**, pp. 25–45.

Chapter 3

Empowerment or Disempowerment: The Limits and Possibilities of Workplace AIDS Policy

David Goss and Derek Adam-Smith

This chapter examines the development and implications of AIDS/HIV policies within organizations as these relate to the treatment of HIV seropositive employees. In Britain, as in many other societies, the advent of HIV and AIDS has always been accompanied by an element of moral panic. The disease was widely perceived as the result of morally questionable behaviour — either male homosexual promiscuity or injecting drug use — and its very potency marked it out in the public imagination as one of the more serious threats of the late twentieth century. While the intensity of this panic has now diminished, it has not disappeared. Indeed, HIV/AIDS continues to pose a substantively different set of problems from other life-threatening or terminal diseases, involving as it does complex layers of meaning, intimately connected with sexuality and morality, with which many people who think of themselves as 'normal' feel distinctly uncomfortable. This situation has been exacerbated by the very novelty of the disease, its sudden 'discovery' and apparently incurable effects: new hazards, especially those for which there is no immediate remedy, generate significant levels of fear and anxiety which, in turn, fuel perceptions of risk (Adam-Smith and Goss, 1993).

In these respects, therefore, HIV/AIDS is dissimilar to many other serious diseases and its occurrence in workplace situations (as in other areas of social life) gives rise to questions which go beyond those posed by other illnesses. In particular, the implications arising from the occurrence of the disease in the workplace can include prejudice against people with HIV/AIDS (manifested in recruitment and promotion discrimination), dismissals (lawful or otherwise), anxiety and fear among employees about contracting the disease, and the 'exposure' of strongly held attitudes about 'legitimate' sexuality (Gutek, 1989). Certainly these questions have often been handled badly by organizations, quite frequently as a result of lack of understanding or ill-informed perceptions of risk and, in many cases simple prejudice, primarily in terms of homophobia but also against those affected by illness (IDS, 1993; Wilson, 1993). Indeed, these prejudices may not be restricted to the employees of a given company, but also extend to customers, clients (including patients) and shareholders (Adam-Smith *et al.*, 1992). Thus, according to the National AIDS Trust:

> [Even] Companies who are models of good practice were reticent about talking to the media. They were worried, and some still are, about how the general public, their shareholders and other companies would react if they associated the company with AIDS.
>
> (National AIDS Trust, 1992: 2)

As an issue, AIDS confronts organizations with the decision whether or not to adopt a positive stance towards people with the disease. In the absence of national or European employment legislation aimed specifically at the protection of people with AIDS, the development of a positive stance is essentially a choice for senior management. Where this choice has been made it usually takes the form of a mission statement coupled to an HIV/AIDS policy.

The context of HIV and AIDS-related organization policy development in the UK has largely been one of piecemeal initiatives based on voluntary rather than statutory principles. The most widely circulated guidance was provided by the Department of Employment and Health and Safety Executive in the 1987 booklet *AIDS and the Workplace*, emphasizing the duty of employers not to discriminate against employees with HIV infection, and to provide education and training for all employees. This has been supplemented by material provided by various public/voluntary sector bodies such as Lesbian and Gay Employment Rights (LAGER, 1990) and local authorities, such as North West Thames Regional Health Authority (1989), usually providing a stronger emphasis on equal opportunities issues. The adoption of policies by UK organizations is difficult to determine with any degree of accuracy due to lack of representative surveys, although evidence from Income Data Services (IDS) (1987; 1993) suggests that policies are more common in the public sector, and in the private sector they are restricted to larger companies. Local studies by Whelan (1992) and Gadd (1993) broadly support this picture. However, the two most sophisticated initiatives focusing on HIV/AIDS and the workplace were launched in 1993 by the National AIDS Trust (NAT) and the Terrence Higgins Trust (THT) respectively. The latter programme, entitled Positive Management, is concerned with protecting employment on the grounds that work, for people with HIV/AIDS, guarantees money and therefore safeguards standard of living. This initiative provides training materials, guidance and a training video based on the good practice of major companies. The NAT scheme, entitled *Companies Act!*, is based on a national charter setting out good practice and encouraging corporate signatories actively to support constructive work in the AIDS field. At the time of writing, there are around twenty-five signatories to the Charter, including companies such as Marks and Spencer, IBM, and National Westminster Bank. The philosophy of *Companies Act!* suggests that 'HIV should be on every personnel manager's agenda; a non-discriminatory policy is the only practical approach. HIV and AIDS are equal opportunities issues, not exclusively health and safety ones' (National AIDS Trust, 1992: 2) The full Guidelines for what constitutes an equitable policy are considered below.

The argument presented below suggests that while the initiatives above represent a generally constructive development, there remain questions as to the operation of HIV/AIDS policies in practice. Thus, although many policies claim to empower employees with HIV/AIDS to enable them to make effective choices about their employment, the success of this objective is likely to be shaped by the general approach to equal opportunities and the culture of the organization concerned. In this respect, simple possession of a constructive HIV/AIDS policy is no guarantee that the potential to empower will be realized. The reasons for this hinge upon two sets of issues. The first relates to the content of AIDS policies and the fact that despite numerous sets of guidelines this is open to widely differing interpretation. The second concerns the common gap between policy and practice and, following from this, the extent to which AIDS policy is actively supported by wider equal opportunities protection. These will be considered in turn.

Policy content

In terms of policy content there are a number of issues that relate strongly to the date of origin of the policy. In particular, we have found a tendency for many documents influenced by the thinking of the 'AIDS panic' of the mid-late 1980s to contain clauses that are factually inaccurate or misleading and to be implicitly or explicitly repressive towards employees with HIV/AIDS. Unfortunately, it seems that many of these policies have not been updated or revised in the light of more recent development. Indeed, on the basis of an analysis of policy documents all obtained within the last two years (although many date back to the late 1980s), we have constructed a distinction between two broad policy approaches: defensive and humanistic (Goss, *et al.*, 1993).[1] This analysis suggests that the substance of policies can vary on two dimensions: *conditionality*, the extent to which the treatment of those with AIDS/HIV is conditional upon (and subordinate to) explicit concerns for organizational interests (either reputation or commercial), and exclusion, the extent to which it is regarded as desirable to identify and separate those with AIDS/HIV either by severance/non-employment or by less favourable treatment.[2]

Those policies which have a high degree of both conditionality and exclusion we have termed *defensive* in that their objective seems to be to retain the maximum room for legal manoeuvre for the organization and the protection of its interests, often at the expense, ultimately, of those with AIDS/HIV.

Defensive policies (implicitly or explicitly) emphasize the potential risk to the organization of employing or continuing to employ someone with AIDS/HIV and prioritize this as the key managerial concern.

On the other hand, those policies which are low on both dimensions we call *humanistic*. These are more concerned to ensure the welfare and protection of the individual and are openly committed to viewing AIDS/HIV both within the workplace and society in terms of social justice and human dignity. Although allowing for the differentiation of individuals with AIDS/HIV where necessary, this is done in a manner which is explicitly non-exclusionary and which guarantees protection if required.

Defensive Policy

Although *defensive policies* have a stated concern to deal fairly with employees who are AIDS 'sufferers' (*sic*) they also contain an assumption that HIV/AIDS poses a threat to workplace operations. In line with much popular reporting of the disease, this type of policy is couched in terms of a defensive response to the threat of attack, with the emphasis upon protecting the (presently) 'healthy' organization from risk. This is often evidenced in references to the damage which could befall the organization should its managers inadvertently con-travene employment laws or generate 'bad publicity'; the implicit emphasis usually being on the consequences of being 'caught out' rather than the ethical nature of the action itself. The following extracts from different policies illustrate this approach[3] (the bulk of policies we have examined come from large private sector employers in both manufacturing and service sectors and from local authorities. S = service sector; M = manufacturing; P = public sector; V = voluntary sector):

> To dismiss an individual who is infected or thought to be infected, because of pressure from work colleagues or the client, may expose us to an *unfair dismissal claim, and furthermore to potentially adverse publicity.* (S)

> Suspension or dismissal solely on the grounds that an employee has become infected is not considered a *practicable* course of action. (M)

> In order to protect our trading position against the risks which can stem from public ignorance and alarm, the PR aspects of individual cases will require careful handling. The prime aim will be to eliminate or at worst minimize publicity in each case. If publicity is unavoidable, the PR department should be asked to advise. (S)

This approach to the issue of HIV/AIDS is reflected in the detailed content of much defensive policy. Where statements relating to the treatment of employees with AIDS are made these are framed in highly conditional terms requiring any action to be assessed against organizational interests, with an implied preference for exclusion where HIV/AIDS is suspected. For example:

> *in general* the company will not dismiss an employee purely on the basis he/she has become infected . . . At this stage medical tests for AIDS are not considered appropriate, unless required by legislation or exceptional *commercial contract arrangements* . . . (Managers) are advised to contact their Personnel department for advice *before contemplating* making a job offer to an AIDS carrier. (S)

> Should an applicant be identified at recruitment as being an AIDS victim or virus carrier, discretion will need to be used as to whether the person should be engaged — depending upon the position being sought, general site circumstances or *other sensitivities believed to be likely to have a bearing on the decision.* (M)

> An employee carrying the HIV virus will be considered for any appointment . . . subject to the same conditions as would apply to any other applicant. The employment prospects of an *employee suffering from AIDS are so limited that such a person would not be considered a suitable candidate for promotion* . . . applications from people suffering from AIDS will not be considered since their work performance and attendance would be *adversely affected by their condition as to make them unsuitable for employment.* (S)

Following this, defensive policy usually provides for mechanisms of surveillance (ranging from testing to reporting procedures of self or others' states of health) designed to identify those with, or suspected of having, HIV/AIDS. As a corollary, considerations of confidentiality and its consequences are given relatively scant regard. Thus:

> In circumstances where it comes to the attention of the unit manager that it is *suspected/*confirmed that we are employing a *potential AIDS suspect*, he/she should immediately notify the Operations Manager. The OM should notify his General Manager Operations, who in turn should notify Personnel and the Regional Director. The RG is responsible for notifying the Divisional Operations Director. (S)

> Should it become known to management that an employee is carrying the HIV virus or suffering from AIDS this information will be held in the strictest confidence and will be made known only to such others as need to know . . . and only with the employee's permission, *except where, permission being withheld, Management concludes, after proper*

> *consideration of all the circumstances . . . that disclosure is necessary in the best interests of the employee, other employees, or the Company.* (S)

> Should you have any fears arising from the behaviour or state of health or any of your fellow employees, you must immediately discuss the matter with your immediate superior. (M)

In summary, then, defensive policy presents HIV/AIDS as a potentially dangerous problem for the organization, the interests of which are prioritized as the standard against which acceptable risk must be assessed.

Humanistic Policy

The impetus behind the development of *humanistic policy* is attributable in no small part to the efforts of AIDS agencies and pressure groups which have fought to safeguard the rights of people with AIDS. Thus the recommendations made by the Companies Act! for an 'equitable AIDS policy' include the following:

- The policy must address both HIV and AIDS separately, and the company's response to each should acknowledge they are separate conditions. HIV and AIDS can be integrated into existing policies, such as those concerning equal opportunities, sickness leave, etc.
- In an integrated policy, mention must be made of HIV and AIDS, to ensure that staff can obtain the information they need on company practice without having to ask specific questions.
- Any policy must clearly state that discrimination, in any aspect of company activity, against anyone who is HIV positive or who has AIDS will not be tolerated.
- The policy should state clearly that AIDS will be treated in the same manner as any other progressive or debilitating illness.
- The policy must contain a clear statement on confidentiality, explaining the way in which confidential information will be treated.
- The policy must make clear, by outlining or referring to discipline and grievance procedures, what action will be taken if staff breach the terms laid down.
- The best model policy will cover areas such as opportunities for redeployment, retraining, flexible working, compassionate leave, etc. Where possible these should apply not only to those infected with HIV but also to carers.

(National AIDS Trust, 1992: Appendix)

In many key respects, therefore, policy based on these principles should exhibit a significantly different emphasis from the Defensive approach. Again this can be illustrated by reference to UK policies we have examined. Consider first the unconditional statements about the treatment of employees with HIV/AIDS:

> There will be no discrimination in recruitment against applicants on the grounds that the applicant has HIV or AIDS. Applicants will not be refused an offer of work because they have AIDS or are anti-body positive. (V)

> Applicants who are deemed to be medically fit at the time of recruitment will not be refused an offer of work because they have AIDS *or* HIV infection. Medical fitness will be determined through the usual process of consideration by the Organization's medical advisers. (P)

Likewise regarding exclusion, this policy stance makes disclosure of HIV status a matter for individual decision and emphasizes the need to avoid unilateral management decisions regarding redeployment (this usually being conditional only upon ability to do the job on medical grounds), placing heavy emphasis on mutual decision-making and respect for individual wishes:

> The Organization has no right to require an individual to disclose that he or she has AIDS or to submit to medical tests for the virus. (P)

> If it becomes known that an employee has AIDS the organization will ensure that resources are available to provide adequate support and any reasonable arrangements to enable work to be continued, on the grounds that to continue working may enable the person to maintain confidence and social contact and fight AIDS with more dignity. (P)

Thus, where differentiation is necessary on medical grounds, care is taken that this is handled in a way which does not result in unfavourable treatment and minimizes the risk of stigmatization. The emphasis is on treating HIV/AIDS as an issue which, in one way or another, involves all employees, requiring positive procedures aimed at encouraging mutual responsibility and support. Indeed, most humanistic policies acknowledge explicitly the assistance of trade unions and/or AIDS agencies in their construction and implementation.

A final distinguishing feature is the role of training and education. Although there is a reliance on information providing techniques (which tend to be factual, 'scientific' and didactic) these are often supplemented by forms of education akin to a community-oriented model involving participatory learning and group work around shared experience. One such seminar run by a private sector organization includes the following issues:

> an understanding of epidemics, sexually transmitted diseases, death, dying, grief, drug use, loss, fear, sexuality, homophobia, prejudice, and

Table 3.1   Contrasting policy approaches to HIV and AIDS

Orientation towards people with AIDS	Defensive policy	Humanistic policy
Language	Conditional; Emphasis on threat and protection; Victim-centred and disempowering	Unconditional; Emphasis on positive image; Empowering
Procedure	Exclusionary; Surveillance; Control	Non-exclusionary; System support
Authority	Primacy of managerial prerogative	Emphasis on consultation; Consent required for most decisions
Training/education	Information-giving model	Information-giving plus community-oriented approaches
Co-operation with extra-organizational bodies.	Minimal, perhaps trade unions informed but not involved at early stages.	Early involvement of trade unions and expert agencies.

the politics and economics of AIDS. Often people have negative attitudes about presumed lifestyles and behaviours. (S)

The key differences between defensive and humanistic policy are summarized in Table 1.

Policy, practice and equal opportunities support

While it is clearly of considerable concern that numerous companies apparently continue to operate with defensive policies, it is likely that with the increased profile of the Positive Management and *Companies Act*! initiatives, the bulk of new organizational policies will tend towards the humanistic position. Certainly we have found no defensive policies formulated after 1990.[4] Even if this is the case, however, there are likely to be many hurdles confronting organizations in making even humanistic policies operate effectively in practice, not the least of which stem from the operation of 'organization sexuality'. It now seems accepted that power tied to sexuality pervades organizations. As Hearn and Parkin put it:

Organisations are characteristically structured and divided both horizontally, in terms of divisions of labour, and vertically, in terms of divisions of authority. These structures do not occur in any abstract way; they occur and are maintained through the social practices of particular people . . . people of similar or different genders and/or sexualities. Thus, we can talk of 'sexual structuring' to refer to these features of organisational structures, in which organisations are continually divided by sex, and indeed sexualities. More precisely we can think of the organisational structuring of sexuality.

(Hearn and Parkin, 1987: 81)

One characteristic of 'organization sexuality' is the dominance of male constructions of heterosexuality over other forms of sexuality (Filby, 1992:24). Indeed, according to Hearn and Parkin:

The dominant concrete form that heterosexuality takes in this society is an hierarchical one. Thus a major, and perhaps central, feature of the sexual 'normality' of organisations is a powerful heterosexual bias: a form of 'compulsory heterosexuality' . . . the domination and oppression of homosexuality, lesbianism and other sexualities perceived as 'other'.

(Hearn and Parkin, 1987: 94)

The recent response of a personnel manager to a course on AIDS-awareness run by a national AIDS charity is probably indicative of the continued tension:

The majority of those who attended the . . . workshop were from public bodies and places of learning. I felt as if I had been hijacked by the AIDS lobby. Everyone in the group was all in favour of equality of sexual practices, and I felt I was in a minority of one seeing homosexuality as an unfortunate aberration and not approving of overt homosexuality . . .

(Johnstone, 1992:45)

A similar attitude, in which the implication of AIDS was apparently raised spontaneously in a discussion of homosexuality, is given by Cockburn :

I asked men [in High Street Retail (one of four case-study firms)] if they thought it would be appropriate to add protection of the employment rights of homosexuals to their equality policy. Few had any inhibitions about voicing a resounding 'no'. 'It's wrong to foster these bent attitudes', 'They are spreading disease — its not good for the nation or for the company' were views widely echoed. Others said, 'I'm not into these bloody weirdos, I just don't want to know', 'It's disgusting, turns my stomach', 'If you want to be "out", it's out *you* go as far as I'm concerned.'

(Cockburn, 1991: 192, emphasis in original)

Indeed, looked at in this light, it does seem that the dominant thrust of humanistic policy is to normalize AIDS, to treat it as 'just another disease', as a means of pre-empting homophobic attack. Thus, whether the policy is freestanding or incorporated into an equal opportunities initiative, the principle concern is with illness rather than sexuality. At one level, this is eminently desirable: the recognition of the work-related health needs of those who have become ill through HIV infection is clearly crucial; similarly, it is undesirable to associate the issue of homosexuality with concerns about illness such that, despite intentions, the former is seen as a cause of the latter. Such normalization is in contrast to the thrust of Defensive policy which is better understood in terms of 'abnormalization' (Goffman, 1963; Burns, 1992) to the extent that it emphasises the difference, 'otherness' and threatening quality of AIDS *per se* and, in so doing, reinforces the 'myth of otherness' and danger which has been attached to those groups directly affected.

At the same time, however, it is also necessary to recognize that, at another level, many of the documented workplace problems associated with AIDS (and also the anecdotal ones) *are* concerned directly with homosexuality and, in this respect, the normalization of HIV infection can mean that, where an organization has no recognition or protection of the rights and entitlements of (in this case) gay men within its other personnel policies and practices, the potential benefits of an HIV/AIDS policy may be partially undermined.

This is because the realization of AIDS policy benefits will (in the UK and in the short-term) hinge disproportionately (although not exclusively) upon the recognition and acceptance of the needs of gay men. In this respect it can be suggested that to be practically effective, AIDS policies need to be supported by, but not directly coupled to, policies on equal opportunities and employee welfare which recognize the legitimacy of a homosexual lifestyle, or which offer rehabilitation and support in the area of substance abuse (Goss, 1993a: 122ff). The reasons for this can be seen in the following areas.

The commitment to non-discrimination

For the non-discrimination aspects of AIDS policy to be effective, the organization must recognize sexual identity as a basis for discrimination as much prejudicial behaviour associated with AIDS will result from homophobia rather than illness. This is well established by anecdotal reports, by industrial tribunal reports and by research findings (e.g. Wilson, 1993; IDS, 1993). In this respect it may be perfectly feasible for an organization member to claim that they are not discriminating on the basis of AIDS or HIV while doing so on the grounds of sexual orientation.

Self-disclosure

Many humanistic policies seek to encourage those who are HIV antibody positive to feel comfortable about voluntarily disclosing their health status in the certainty that their employment prospects will be protected, their confidentiality secured and their medical needs met effectively should this arise. However, without wider protection of rights this runs the risk of making access problematic for those who feel that their illness will be linked to some other factor — homosexuality or drug use — that they fear will not receive such sympathetic treatment. Some evidence to support this would seem to be provided by Keay and Leach (1993) who claim that HIV/AIDS is not an issue that arises in personal counselling provided by employers.

Bereavement

The principal area of welfare where sexual orientation will make a difference is in relation to compassionate leave. Here it will be necessary for the organization to recognize the responsibilities and commitments of gay men towards their (ill) partners and their right to bereavement leave, etc. At present many organizations, if they provide such benefits at all, operate with a narrow and conventional (i.e. heterosexual) view of family and close relatives.

Thus, where an organization is uneasy about the issue of sexual orientation, there may also be a tendency for an HIV/AIDS policy, while accepted in theory, to be neutralized in practice. This will usually mean locating the policy strictly as a health or medical issue. We have come across a number of organizations, both public and private sector, that have been developing AIDS policies but have decided to locate these within the health and safety remit as a means of ensuring that it could not be interpreted as condoning homosexuality which was perceived as being an issue that would be politically unpopular at local level or likely to cause problems with the board.

Conclusions

Following the work of Herek and Glunt (1991) on AIDS-related attitudes, we have developed a tentative typology of organizational reactions to AIDS. Herek and Glunt's US research labels the axes of the typology *pragmatism/moralism* (corresponding to our abnormalizing/normalizing) and *coercion/compassion*

```
                          LONG AGENDA
                        (Equal Opportunities)
                                 │
        Empowering               │     Inconsistent
    (Compassionate secularism)   │   (Indiscriminate action)
                                 │
                                 │
NORMALIZING ─────────────────────┼───────────────── ABNORMALIZING
(Humanistic policy)              │              (Defensive policy)
                                 │
        Neutralising             │     Disempowering
    (Compassionate moralism)     │    (Punitive moralism)
                                 │
                          SHORT AGENDA
                        (Equal Opportunities)
```

Figure 3.1   A tentative typology of organizational responses to AIDS

(corresponding to our long agenda/short agenda) and define their quadrants (given in parentheses in our typology) as follows.

> First, the Compassionate Secularism pattern characterises the general stance of the American public health community and of the lesbian and gay male community: endorsement of such non-moralistic pragmatic policies as distribution of condoms and sterile needles, as well as opposition to coercive measures such as quarantine . . . Second, a pattern of Compassionate Moralism . . . is reflected in the official pronouncements of the Conference of Catholic Bishops: compassion is urged for people with AIDS, but education about condoms is rejected on moral grounds . . . Third, Punitive Moralism, endorsement of coercive measures and rejection of non-moralistic pragmatic policies, is perhaps best exemplified in the US by spokespersons of conservative political and religious beliefs . . . Indiscriminate Action . . . may reflect an acquiescent response set (and) considerable ambivalence concerning AIDS: views of people with AIDS as both dangerous and deserving of compassion . . . containment as well as pragmatic education and prevention.
>
> (Cited in Pollak, 1992: 28)

In our typology we use Cockburn's (1991) distinction between long and short equal opportunities agendas for the vertical access and the previously developed concepts of normalizing and abnormalizing policy for the horizontal.

Thus *Disempowering* responses represent attempts to exclude those with (or perceived to be associated with) HIV/AIDS from the organization by means of dismissal (lawful or unlawful) and /or intimidation (these attitudes are represented in several of the industrial tribunal cases in the UK where HIV/

AIDS has been an issue and in the cases described by Wilson, 1993). *Inconsistent* responses are likely to operate where there is a gap between a generalized commitment to equality of opportunity and a policy that is substantively unable to deliver constructive treatment of people with HIV/AIDS. The result may be practices that are contradictory and prone to cynical manipulation. *Neutralizing* responses reflect attempts to treat HIV/AIDS as just another disease but fail to recognize (or deliberately deny) that it raises, either directly or indirectly, issues of equality of opportunity. Finally, *Empowering* approaches offer the prospect of dealing constructively with the practical/medical workplace needs of people with HIV/AIDS at the same time as providing a separate and comprehensive commitment to equal opportunities based on minority rights *per se*.

Although there is evidence for the existence of these different types of organizational responses provided by our own ongoing research and by secondary source material, the as yet incomplete nature of our findings means that we present this typology only as a provisional starting point for discussion and further exploration rather than as a definitive statement. In particular, we would note that there is a dual potential attached to the notion of normalization (one offers the possibility of empowerment, the other, in the Foucauldian sense, a form of control and discipline). Crucially, however, it is likely that for the empowering potential of normalization to be realized, it will be necessary for there to be *independent* equal opportunities support based on a long agenda. Where this is not present, it is unlikely that HIV policies, no matter how carefully constructed, will realize their full potential for empowerment nor appear as user-friendly to that group most likely to have need of them.

Despite these misgivings, this is not an argument against policies. Certainly, our research suggests that policy can have an important educative and procedural role to play in terms of general awareness, health education and good practice (Adam-Smith and Goss, 1993; Gadd, 1993). To the extent that this activity may indirectly empower employees affected by HIV/AIDS by increasing levels of understanding and support, it is to be welcomed (Goss, 1993b). To be fully empowering, however, may need more than a good AIDS policy alone.

Notes

1 Thus far the project has examined 20 policies in the original, and a further 30 from secondary sources. Of those policies we have examined the ratio of *defensive* to *humanistic* is in the order of 1:5. This may be a reflection of a greater preparedness of organizations with humanistic policies, knowing these to be 'good practice' to allow outside disclosure.
2 Initial inspection of the policy documents indicated a number of points of variation which gave rise to two sets of 'grounded' concepts: *conditionality* and *exclusion*.

Conditionality captures the extent to which the treatment of those with HIV/AIDS is defined as conditional upon explicit concerns for organizational interests (either reputation or commercial) and reflects the following policy dimensions.

(a) The origin of the statements. Here there were three discernible patterns: first, policies written by and/or for a specific organization (bespoke); second, those which followed a standardized form and content, usually based on government or sector guidelines (off-the-peg); and finally, hybrid policies which combined off-the-peg elements with bespoke additions.

(b) The construction of the policy. This is related to the way in which policy statements have been organized. For example, does an off-the-peg policy contain all the elements of the original text or only some parts? Which off-the-peg elements do hybrids adopt and how are these related to bespoke aspects? In particular, to what extent does the (re)construction of the policy reflect an attempt to (re)define nondiscrimination statements through the insertion of conditional clauses relating to organizational interests?

Exclusion is indicated by the extent to which a policy provides for the (detrimental) identification and separation of those with HIV/AIDS either by severance/non-employment or by less favourable treatment.

(a) The substantive content. There was variation in the extent to which the policies embodied specific procedural and rule-based frameworks and, more importantly, in the ways in which these prioritized either the interests of those with HIV/AIDS or those of the organization. This would relate to issues of disclosure and control of health state, confidentiality of such information, and procedures for handling discovered cases of HIV/AIDS.

(b) The language and tone of the policy. Here there were differences in the extent to which policies used language which was either stigmatizing or victim-centred.

3 Confidentiality assurances prevent us from naming the companies involved other than by sector. Each quoted extract in both *defensive* and *humanistic* categories is taken from a separate policy. All emphases are added by us.

4 In order to extend our research on organizational implications of HIV/AIDS we are currently undertaking a survey of organizations in South East England and an extensive interview programme across regions and industrial sectors. The survey investigates policy steps taken to deal with HIV/AIDS. Two hundred and fifty randomly selected private sector businesses in Hampshire, Sussex and Dorset were sent questionnaires yielding a 24 per cent response rate. The interview programme, sponsored by ESRC, involves detailed semi-structured interviews with a cross-section of organization members in 15 (non-randomly selected) organizations in public, private and voluntary sectors, yielding a total of 150 interviews. In both cases, the data has only been subject to preliminary analysis and the ideas expressed in this section must be regarded as tentative and provisional. However, results from the survey do suggest some grounds for optimism in the development of constructive AIDS policy to the extent that most of the managers who responded appeared to have a reasonably good factual knowledge of HIV/AIDS (Adam-Smith and Goss, 1993; Gadd, 1993) and felt it to be an issue that *ought* to be handled in a constructive and equitable manner. However, there was also uncertainty about whether this could be achieved in practice. This ambivalence has been reflected in the interview programme, where there appears to be an emerging disjunction between what employees claim to feel as individuals, how they perceive the feelings of others in the organization, and how they think the organization expects them to behave in dealing with HIV/AIDS issues. In particular, a key issue in this concern appears to be homosexuality, which they perceive as being linked inextricably to HIV/AIDS in most people's minds. An emerging response involves the assertion that although they themselves are not prejudiced, other organization members are perceived to be less tolerant (either through ignorance or bigotry). Thus, senior managers are often claimed to view a

public association with AIDS and homosexuality as threatening the organization's image, whereas lower level employees are presumed to harbour (media-induced) prejudices against homosexuals, and would therefore see an AIDS policy as offering support and favouritism to an undeserving group.

References

ADAM-SMITH, D. and GOSS, D. (1993) 'HIV/AIDS and the hospitality industry: Some implications of perceived risk', *Employee Relations*, Special edition, **15**, 2.

ADAM-SMITH D., GOSS, D., SINCLAIR, A., RESPONSES, G. and MEUDELL, K. (1992) 'AIDS and Employment: diagnosis and prognosis', *Employee Relations*, **18**, 3, pp. 29–40.

BURNS, T. (1992) *Erving Goffman*, London: Routledge.

COCKBURN, C. (1991) *In the Way of Women*, London: Macmillan.

FILBY, M. (1992) 'The Figures, the personality and the bums: Service work and sexuality', *Work Employment and Society*, **6, 1**, pp. 23–42.

GADD, K. (1993) 'Report to Portsmouth AIDS forum (unpublished), Centre for AIDS and Employment Research', Portsmouth: Portsmouth Business School.

GOFFMAN, E. (1963) *Stigma*, Harmondsworth: Penguin Books.

GOSS, D. (1993a) *Principles of Human Resource Management*, London: Routledge.

GOSS, D. (1993b) 'Moral dilemmas and moral issues: The ethical implications of HIV/AIDS', *Business Ethics: a European Journal*, **2**, 3, pp. .143–48.

GOSS, D., ADAM-SMITH, D., SINCLAIR, A. and RESPONSES, G. (1993) 'AIDS policies as data: possibilities and precautions', *Sociology*, **27**, 2, pp. 299–305.

GUTEK, B. (1989) 'Sexuality in the workplace: Key issues in social research and organisation practice', in HEARN, J., SHEPPARD, D., TANCRED-SHERIFF, P. and BURRELL, G. (Eds) *The Sexuality of Organisation*, London: Sage.

HEARN, J. and PARKIN, W. (1987) *Sex at Work: the Power and Paradox of Organisation Sexuality*, Brighton: Wheatsheaf.

HEREK, G. and GLUNT, E. (1991) 'AIDS-related attitudes in the US', *Journal of Sex Research*, **28**, 1, pp. 99–123.

IDS (1987) *AIDS and Employment*, Incomes Data Services Study 393.

IDS (1993) *AIDS returns to the Agenda*, Incomes Data Services Study 528.

JOHNSTONE, V. (1992) 'How should we respond to AIDS?', *Sunday Telegraph*, 29 March, p. 45.

KEAY, D. and LEACH, M. (1993) 'Positive thinking about HIV', *Human Resources*, Spring, pp. 36–40.

LAGER (1990) *HIV and AIDS: Policy Guidelines for Voluntary Organisations and Small Employers*, London: Lesbian and Gay Employment Rights.

NATIONAL AIDS TRUST (1992) *Companies Act! The Business Charter on HIV/AIDS*, London: National AIDS Trust.

NW THAMES REGIONAL HEALTH AUTHORITY (1989) *HIV Infection and the Workplace*, London: NW Thames HIV Project.

POLLAK, M. (1992) 'Attitudes, beliefs and opinions in POLLAK, M., PAICHELER, G. and PIERRET, J. *AIDS: A Problem for Sociological Research*, London: Sage.

WHELAN, S. (1992) *Managing a Crisis? Employer Policy in HIV/AIDS in North Nottinghamshire*, North Nottinghamshire Health Authority.

WILSON, P. (1993) *HIV and AIDS in the Workplace*, London: National AIDS Trust.

Chapter 4

Outreach, Community Change and Community Empowerment: Contradictions for Public Health and Health Promotion

Tim Rhodes

In Britain, the HIV epidemic has encouraged a rapid revision in policy approaches to drug treatment and prevention, characterized by the emergence of pragmatism (Stimson, 1990; Stimson and Lart, 1991). This has encompassed increased recognition of the importance of community-based responses to HIV-related prevention, treatment and care (Advisory Council on the Misuse of Drugs (ACMD) 1988; 1989; 1993) and of the impracticality of an absolutist reliance on abstentionist oriented medical and legal interventions in reducing the health-related harms associated with illicit drug use (O'Hare *et al.*, 1992).

The shift towards pragmatism in HIV prevention has facilitated the development of what have come to be viewed as innovative styles of service delivery. These have been characterized by user friendly communication philosophies promising low threshold access to drug treatment and HIV prevention (Hart *et al.*, 1989). The implementation of a nationwide network of syringe exchange schemes and the rapid development of extra-agency initiatives such as detached outreach work have come to be viewed as key components of a wider public health HIV prevention strategy (Stimson *et al.*, 1991; Rhodes and Hartnoll, 1991).

For some, the development of outreach has been viewed as a long awaited panacea in the race to reach the hardest-to-reach drug injectors. For others there is as much to criticize as there is to celebrate. While outreach may have much to offer as a harm reduction strategy and as a method of HIV prevention, its demonstrated successes are sometimes eclipsed by its manifest limitations. By considering the limitations of outreach as a method of health education for injecting drug users, it is possible to appraise critically the current and future role of outreach in the public health prevention of HIV infection among drug injectors and their sexual and sharing partners. It also becomes possible to explicate the potential contradictions between community health approaches and public health perspectives with regard to the facilitation of empowerment over health and health choices among drug injectors and their peers.

The promise of health promotion and the new public health

The *new* public health, of which a comprehensive and integrated health promotion is a part, advocates the need to balance individual and collective action as a means of facilitating and enabling changes in individual and collective health status (Nutbeam and Blakey, 1990; Ashton and Seymour, 1990; Bunton and Macdonald, 1992). The new public health movement of the 1980s promised to move beyond a bio-medical understanding of health and illness towards a new understanding of social action which encompasses the social and environmental influences on health, health choices and health behaviour. Health promotion thereby came to be re-defined as the intersectoral activity which aims to enable individuals and communities to increase control over the factors which influence and improve their health (Tannahill, 1985; Nutbeam, 1986; Bunton and Macdonald, 1992). This demands an integrated and comprehensive health promotion practice, such as that outlined in the World Health Organization *Ottawa Charter for Health Promotion* (WHO, 1986; Nutbeam and Blakey, 1990).

The Ottawa Charter, which provides a framework for the promotion of health, identifies the need for intervention strategies to develop individual personal, social and political skills; re-orients health services towards the objective of health gain; facilitates and strengthens community action; creates supportive and healthy environments; and promotes public policy supportive of health (WHO, 1986). In essence, these five principles can be summarized as healthy individuals; healthy services; healthy communities; healthy environments; and healthy policy (Rhodes, 1994a). While the Ottawa Charter principles are supportive of the ideal of an *integrated* approach to health promotion, they are also the source of theoretical and practical conflict in defining, justifying and prioritizing health promotion activity (Beattie, 1986; 1991). Indeed, they form a hierarchy of ideals which are as *political* in their meaning and implications for change as they are practical.

Health promotion and the new public health may have many promises, but they also have many failures. The advocacy of strategies for community, environmental and political action is clearly very different from an application of these strategies. With regard to the new public health and the development of harm reduction strategies for drug services, Stimson and Lart (1991) have described these promises as 'new words' and the practices as 'old tunes'. When considering health promotion and the development of outreach as a method of community-based HIV prevention, the outcome is similar: there is little reality in the rhetoric.

The challenge for HIV-prevention services is to move from the *advocacy* of health promotion towards its *application* (Rhodes, 1994a). This need is most explicit where prevention and harm reduction activity is most essential; among harder-to-reach individuals and communities who have an inequity of access to health and health services (Rhodes and Holland, 1992). It is here also that the inherent contradictions between public health (new and old) and community health perspectives become most evident. The evolution and development of outreach as a method of HIV prevention provides a useful and incisive instance of this process.

This chapter aims to consider the limitations and possibilities of outreach as a strategy of HIV-related health promotion among harder-to-reach drug injectors. In doing so, it considers the developments and dilemmas associated with some key concepts much favoured and oft advocated in community-based HIV prevention work. These include the notions of empowerment, community change and community organization. In critically examining the practical and theoretical utility of these concepts, potential developments in the future direction and focus of outreach can be identified.

Outreach Promises, Outreach Practices: The Limits of Individualism

Like the new public health movement, within which present day community development interventions can be located, HIV outreach appears to have as many promises as it has failures. It is clear that as a mode of health education, outreach has much to offer. It is an extra agency response which aims to reach those most in need of health services with the objective of facilitating change directly in the community (Rhodes and Hartnoll, 1991). It has the capacity to intervene within the everyday social realities of drug users' lifestyles and behaviours. Whereas most prevention work amongst injecting drug users remains confined to the office — as does the *impact* of many prevention messages — outreach promises to go further. It promises to reach out in response to need and to create the possibilities for change.

Not all promises are fulfilled. As indicated in recent evaluation work, current outreach remains demonstrably weak in identifying and responding to consumer need and considerably limited in its ability to demonstrate healthy behaviour change (Rhodes and Holland, 1992). As recently described by McDermott, outreach *promises* do not necessarily equate with outreach *practices*:

> Starved of effective supervision, many workers spend more time in the office, at conferences or in the ubiquitous 'meetings', than they do in the streets. Others sit around in the homes of existing contacts, or provide a

free taxi service for drug users, rather than reaching out and making new contacts

(McDermott, 1993:13)

Current outreach for drug injectors remains limited in scope for reaching and responding to consumer need and in facilitating changes in the community (Rhodes, 1993; Stimson *et al.*, 1994). UK outreach has been characterized by practically rather than theoretically driven interventions and by an inhibited theoretical framework which constrains the possibilities for change. This theoretical framework does not have a vocabulary for the community or for the collective but is instead characterised and limited by individualism.

First, outreach is inherently limited in the extent to which it is able to reach potential consumers. Because outreach focuses on contacting individuals on a one-to-one worker-client basis 'it allows only arithmetic progression into the target population, limiting the numbers who can be effectively reached' (Stimson, *et al.*, 1994) While it is clearly ridiculous for outreach workers to reach *every* individual within a specified target population, it is equally questionable whether outreach has been effective in reaching the *appropriate* individuals. Evaluation shows that many of the easier to reach individuals contacted by outreach are probably less in need of such services than those who remain hidden to even the most skilled or streetwise of outreach workers (Rhodes and Holland, 1992). For some, many outreach services 'are failing to make and maintain contact with injecting drug users' (McDermott, 1993:13).

Second, current outreach is limited by the methods and strategies it commonly employs to facilitate change. By far the majority of outreach interventions are client-centred in that they target *individuals* with the aim of achieving *self-empowerment* over health choices and health status. Quite apart from the brevity and the style of the contact, the language of self-empowerment and self-enablement is limited. Not only is it often paternalistic and even patronizing, it fails to recognize that individual choices about health or risk may not actually be choices at all. For outreach providers and consumers alike, individual perceptions and understandings of risk, and individual control over *choice* with regard to health and health behaviour, are relative both to wider peer group, social and community norms and to situational and material conditions (Friedman *et al.*, 1990; Bloor *et al.*, 1992; Grund *et al.*, 1992; Romer and Hornik, 1992).

The notion of self-empowerment assumes the appropriate supportive social and material conditions in which individuals can exercise choice. In practice, this means individual empowerment approaches are often only partially effective, ranging from the informed choice to the informed *no* choice, but rarely enabling a *free* choice. Just as outreach providers are unable to simply choose safer sex in the same way as they might a toothpaste, neither can (or should) they expect consumers of outreach services to be in a position to choose healthier lifestyles.

Behaviours attributed risky by the epidemiologist are part of a wider structure or culture of behaviours, which participants often view and experience as normal, rational, even mundane (Schwartz and Jacobs, 1979; Stimson, 1992). This means individual empowerment — and the related concepts of self-assertion, self-esteem and self-efficacy — have limited capabilities for understanding and influencing the social realities of everyday behaviours deemed risky or unhealthy. In response, outreach needs to consider the possibilities for facilitating changes or endorsements in everyday peer group and community norms about health and health behaviour, with the objective of creating the social conditions necessary for individual change (Rhodes, 1993).

The limits of individualism in community-based responses to harm reduction and HIV prevention are noted by Stimson *et al.* (1991) in the context of evaluation of syringe exchange. They note that the syringe exchange model is inherently limited in encouraging and sustaining changes among drug injectors directly in the community. This is because the sharing of injecting equipment is influenced not by availability alone but by situational context, by the dynamics of particular social relationships, and by social desirability and acceptability (McKeganey and Barnard, 1992; Burt and Stimson, 1993). Ethnographic work, for example, shows that while the social etiquette of injecting drug use has changed and that while needle and syringe sharing is considered less the norm by drug injectors (Burt and Stimson, 1993), sharing continues to occur within particular social networks of injectors under certain social and situational conditions where different norms and values prevail (Murphy, 1987; McKeganey and Barnard, 1992).

Future outreach promises: from the individual to the collective

In recent years there has been increasing advocacy of outreach which aims to change the peer group and community norms and behaviours that influence and sustain individual unhealthy behaviours (Friedman *et al.*, 1992; Friedman, de Jong and Wodak, 1993). This introduces the possibility of interventions oriented not towards individuals but towards social networks and communities. Recent debates in health promotion have characterized a number of theoretically distinct types of health education practice, which range from self empowerment approaches, to community action and socially transformatory or radical-political approaches (Beattie, 1991; Draper *et al.*, 1980; Homans and Aggleton, 1988). Following these models, client-centred outreach favouring self-empowerment can be seen as *individual* outreach while community-oriented or population-oriented outreach can be seen as *community* outreach (Stimson *et al.*, 1994). Community outreach thus aims to encourage community change in peer group and community norms and behaviours (Rhodes, 1993; 1994b). As recommended in the latest report of the Advisory Council on the Misuse of Drugs, *AIDS and Drugs Misuse*, 'Achieving community change should be the focus of outreach work at least as much as securing individual change' (ACMD, 1993:4.16).

A community outreach perspective needs to employ intervention methods designed to overcome the limits of individualism described above. As has been suggested elsewhere, those most effective in achieving community change are drug users themselves (Wiebel, 1988). Following the principles of *community action* in health promotion which involves 'deliberate organization of community members to accomplish some objective or goal' (Brown, 1991:446), peer education has proved both feasible and effective in facilitating community-based change.

In a number of outreach interventions in the United States, client driven and indigenous leader models of outreach employ current or former drug users as peer educators (prevention advocates) to pass on socially responsible beliefs and health recommendations to their drug injecting friends and peers (NIDA, 1989; Wiebel, 1988; Broadhead *et al.*, 1993). Research has found peer influence and endorsement to be an important determinant of drug-related behaviour changes, as well as sexual behaviour changes among drug injectors and their sexual partners (Abdul-Quadar *et al.*, 1990, 1992; Tross *et al.*, 1992; Sotheran *et al.*, 1989; Friedman *et al.*, 1991). More particularly, research has shown interventions using peer education and norm-changing methods to be more effective than individually-focused outreach and health education alone (Grund *et al.*, 1992; Friedman *et al.*, 1992; Kelly *et al.*, 1991, 1992).

This approach, which is oriented towards networks or communities, introduces the wider — and stronger — notion of *community empowerment*. This encourages mobilization towards collective ownership and control over health choices and health status. Following the relative success of community development and mobilization interventions within gay communities, this has led to attempts to organize drug injectors and their peers (Friedman *et al.*, 1992; Friedman, de Jong and Wodak, 1993). The use of peer influence as a method of initiating and reinforcing change in drug injectors' social and health relationships can be viewed as the first step towards a process of community and collective change. It may also be considered the first step towards providing the foundation for mobilization and organization of drug injectors. *Community organization*, which in health promotion involves 'any effort to form temporary or permanent organisational structures involving members of a community' (Brown, 1991:446), thus aims to enable community empowerment towards defining and controlling collective norms and values about health, and in confronting the wider social and material constraints which marginalize equity to a public health issue.

Community and community change: political and practical

The term *community* has gained much currency in public health and health promotion discourse. But despite much talk of *communities* and of *community* change, the notion of community is problematic (Patton, 1990). A definition and understanding of community is clearly central to the planning and targeting of community-based interventions, particularly those advocating community change. Not only has the Advisory Council on the Misuse of Drugs (ACMD) emphasized the importance of community-based intervention in the care, treatment and prevention of HIV and drug-related problems (ACMD, 1988; 1989), it has also endorsed the idea of the community itself acting as an agent for change (ACMD, 1993). It is clear that the nature and structure of communities both help and inhibit the conditions and possibilities for change (Rogers and Shoemaker, 1971; Tones, Tilford and Robinson, 1990). It is also clear that health promoters differ widely in their definition and usage of the term. As noted by Rose (1990), the only thing the term often has in common is that it is about people.

In health promotion, a community has been 'distinguished from any other social aggregation in respect of its relative size, geographical contiguity and the nature of the social network and norms prevailing within this circumscribed locality' (Tones, Tilford and Robinson, 1990:235). This introduces a number of key factors central to defining or circumscribing a body of people as a *community*: size, geography, social network dynamics and social norms. Historically, community development has targeted geographically defined communities where 'the propinquity of the inhabitants has relevance for those interests or needs which they share' (Calouste Gulbenkian Foundation, 1984). In health promotion practice, these communities have been viewed as population catchment areas as large as 20 000 (Henderson and Thomas, 1980). While locality or geography may be of some importance in targeting community outreach among a network of drug injectors, it is clear that this is not likely to be the only or the key determining factor. It may be of more benefit to conceive of the nature of drug injecting social networks in terms of their *differentiation, centrality* and *solidarity* (MacCannell, 1979) with regard to the prevailing norms, beliefs and behaviours within them. This, however, does not simply explain or determine when a group of drug injectors can be usefully or easily circumscribed as a community. Equally importantly, it raises the question of who defines drug injecting social networks as communities and whether drug injectors identify themselves as such. This in turn raises questions about the rhetoric of community as a political formation as opposed to a social reality.

Community: Political Formation or Social Reality?

For some the term *community* carries with it a package of ostensibly political meanings and objectives. For others the term is rather mundane. While for the health activist, community is integral to wider discourses of political organization, for the health interventionist (and for health promotion) community is ostensibly a socially — rather than politically — organized and circumscribed constitutency.

The language of community is double-edged. On the one hand, it can serve the purpose of designating groups of individuals which are collectively distinct and disenfranchised from larger society, and on the other, it can serve the purposes of blurring or erasing these structural demarcations and inequalities (Horton, 1989; Patton, 1990). For Horton, the concept of community is most useful when it recognizes that communities are 'not necessarily pre-given but are often forged through the collective experience of oppression to which they respond' (Horton, 1989:173). Following this usage, it is argued that the term community is inappropriately applied when attached to dominant hegemonic sections of society, such as the heterosexual community, the European Community or the international community. This is because such an application of the term community serves to blur the social realities of structural inequalities which have helped shape collectively distinct communities and subcultures. Community in this restricted sense — is a *political* formation (Patton, 1990) cognizant with a health activism which concomitantly recognizes the ideological dominance of professionalized and medicalized health services and the need to address health inequalities through empowerment of the disenfranchised and marginalized. The notion of community can therefore be politically empowering in that it can encourage shared and distinct identity and values among disenfranchised or marginalized populations in the context of wider society's attempts to homogenise and eradicate such difference (Patton, 1990).

While this may be so, it remains questionable the extent to which such a notion of community fits the social realities of injecting drug use and of drug injecting social networks. Just as the notion of *heterosexual community* can be co-opted as a method of blurring the structural imbalances and differences of identity within, so can the notion of a *disenfranchised* community blur the intra-social realities of injecting drug use and sexual practices:

> the meanings of sexuality or drug use are engendered within networks of face-to-face communication and within cultural productions . . . which *cut across* the 'communities' articulated for the purpose of engaging in the political languages of civil rights and claims for apportionment of social resources
>
> (Patton, 1990:8)

This is particularly so with regard to drug users and drug-using social networks. While research points to the importance of community mobilization and community identity in creating the social and cultural conditions necessary for sexual behaviour change among gay men (Watney, 1990; Kippax *et al.*, 1992; Kelly *et al.*, 1991a, 1992), the facilitation of community participation and a community identity among drug users is more problematic and may be inappropriate. This is because the social relationships which frame many drug using activities tend to be predatory rather than participative, functional rather than ideological (Rhodes, 1993). While research has demonstrated the normative importance of sharing in drug users' social and material relationships (McKeganey and Barnard, 1992), and of peer influence in supporting and sustaining changes in drug use and sexual behaviour (see above), such norms and social relationships may not be experienced or understood as part of a *community* identity. The notion of community lacks both the specificity and applicability to account fully for, or to encourage, changes in drug users' social relationships.

With regard to facilitating safer sexual practices, these problems are particularly acute. It is possible to envisage safer sex as community practice among gay communities (Watney, 1990) because the social construction of gay community identity overlaps with the social realities of sexuality and sexual practice. Among drug injecting networks, while it is possible to envisage the use of clean works as community practice, it becomes more difficult to envisage a shared social responsibility or community identity about safer sex and sexuality. The construction of community identity among drug injectors in the light of sexual health promotion poses additional problems as sexual practices and sexuality do not enjoy 'master status'. In short, the currency of drug injecting social networks are largely based on the shared knowledge and practices of injecting drug use rather than those of sex and sexuality.

While marginalized and disenfranchized from larger society, it is far more likely that drug injecting networks are sustained because of functional need (dealing, scoring and using drugs) than they are because of the collective experience of oppression to which Horton refers. Indeed, recent ethnographic research in London (Power and Jones, 1993) tends to suggest that social networks of drug injectors are characterized by less *Gemeinschaft* (interpersonal interactions) than they are *Gesellschaft* (impersonal interactions). This suggests that the notion of community as a political formation has less of an immediate practical utility among drug injectors than among some other sub-populations where there exists a shared sense of social and political identity and where infrastructures for action already exist (Patton, 1990).

Following Becker's work on the social organization of drug-related knowledge and the emergence of collective identity and subculture (Becker, 1963, 1967b), it is useful to view emergent communities of drug injectors in the light of shared networks of knowledge, experience and behaviour. This is not to deny the existence or the possibility of a shared social, political or community identity among drug injectors. It does, however, allow for the possibilities and realities of peer health education and community change among drug-injecting networks in the context of there often existing little political or collective identity within them. The role of community outreach in this context is to understand the homogeneity (and heterogeneity) of shared norms, beliefs and behaviour within and across social networks of drug injectors. The community — from an interventionist perspective — can be practically defined as 'a set of formal or informal relationships that has some established criteria for membership'

(Amsel, 1990). It is the task of outreach to view these relationships as 'the everyday shared norms, values and practices relevant for change or endorsement when targeting modifications in health behaviour (Rhodes, 1993:1318).

This means that community change among drug injecting social networks can occur without these groupings necessarily defining or identifying themselves as a community. This is clearly a weaker conception of community — particularly in the context of political and activist organizing (see below) — but it provides an intermediate target for intervention in encouraging community change and — over time — community organization. Viewing the notion of community in this way allows interventionists to view and target particular social networks of drug injectors as communities with the aim of either *introducing* and facilitating community identity and practices, or of *strengthening* pre-existing identity and practices. The latter is clearly the more powerful, but both share the broader aim of making the communities of political rhetoric, one and the same as the communities of social reality.

Community empowerment: whose side are you on?

The idea of community empowerment is useful in conceptualizing peer education and community change interventions as distinct from those targeting individuals and self-empowerment. However, the concept may be of limited practical use in understanding or describing the social realities of health promotion practice among drug injectors and their sexual/sharing partners. While health promotion and the new public health promises empowerment, there remain fundamental theoretical and practical contradictions between community health and public health approaches. These contradictions — made explicit in the context of HIV prevention and injecting drug use — are both political and practical.

Empowerment necessarily means the displacing of power in practice (Tones, 1986). This necessitates questioning critically the values of those in power. In the context of public and community health intervention, this demands questioning the concepts of *healthy* and *unhealthy* and the extent to which marginalized individuals and communities have an equity of *choice* over these values. As said by Howard Becker on the subject of values in social science research, 'The question is not whether we should take sides, since we inevitably will, but rather whose side are we on?' (Becker, 1967a:239)

Community outreach in the United Kingdom is still more rhetoric than reality. Despite this, it is important to question how likely it is that the future promises of outreach will become the future practices of outreach. While peer education and community action approaches may be effective in achieving change among social networks of drug injectors, this may be quite distinct from achieving community empowerment. It is unlikely that empowerment will be achieved by facilitating and supporting changes in peer group norms and behaviours alone. This is particularly the case with regard to a relatively disenfranchized or marginalized social group such as drug injectors, despite their degree of internal community solidarity or cohesiveness. Because empowerment means the displacing of social, political and material power in practice, community empowerment remains problematic among drug injecting social networks given that such groupings remain *dis*-empowered *sub*communities.

While health promotion promises to work 'through collective community action' with 'communities having their own power and having control of their own initiatives and activities' (Ashton and Seymour, 1990:26), this is rarely attempted and hardly ever achieved (Brown, 1991; Farrant, 1991). Among drug injecting networks across the world, there is increasing advocacy of community development, participation and organization (Friedman, de Jong and Wodak, 1993; Friedman *et al.*, 1992; Burrows and Price, 1993). These vary from alliances between current and former drug injectors and interested health professionals to — increasingly — collectively run groups and organizations of drug injectors. To a varying extent, these organizations take as their aims not only changes in community norms and behaviours but also changes in wider social, political and material conditions. Community organizing is not only community action, it is also political action; it aims to achieve not only healthy *communities*, but social and political change and healthy *policy*.

Community organizing initiatives among drug injecting networks have much to learn from the experiences and successes of AIDS organizing and AIDS activism within gay communities (Crimp, 1988; Patton, 1990). There remain, however, fundamental contradictions in the language and practices of community development when applied to the social realities of organizing among drug injectors, particularly where social networks have little notion of community identity or solidarity. While it is both possible and necessary to encourage the consumers of outreach services to become the providers of outreach services in the form of peer educators, this is very different from drug injectors themselves owning and controlling the aims, objectives and practices of intervention. Peer education and community change interventions are clearly the next step towards outreach approaches but these — in themselves — cannot achieve community empowerment. This can only be achieved when drug injectors themselves have collective ownership and control over what is healthy and unhealthy and over choices with regard to HIV-related behaviour and (ultimately) HIV transmission.

This highlights potential contradictions between community health and public health approaches. Quite apart from the possibilities or realities of drug injecting networks being empowered with regard to health choices (or any other social, welfare or material issue), community empowerment allows communities to make choices which other (more dominant) communities may consider unhealthy to the public health (Labonte, 1989; Tones, 1986). This is because the new public health presumes a rationality of choice-making which makes 'healthy choices the *rational* choices' (Thorogood, 1992). The new public health thus comprises a political and moral agenda, for it can not allow empowered wrong choices to be right, healthy or rational. Indeed, as suggested by Labonte, 'what communities do for their own health may be inimical to public health' (Labonte, 1989:87) and as suggested by Brown, 'health professionals have a responsibility to voice their own views and values and not blindly or slavishly support the community' (Brown, 1991:452).

Drawing on Becker's notion of a 'hierarchy of credibility' of values and value-making (Becker, 1967a), it is clear that public health professionals and providers define what is healthy and unhealthy. Equally importantly, they define what is *public*. This means that the progressive and increasingly favoured rhetoric of free choice and community empowerment can amount to false promises of the new public health movement. Peer education can thus equate to peer manipulation if those from outside drug injecting communities are manipulating choices about what is healthy and what is unhealthy. The 'single rationality' offered by public health (Thorogood, 1992) compromises what might be considered true community-development because it implicitly homogenizes difference into sameness: rather than empowering real choice for the consumer, it offers the illusion of choice.

It is for this reason that the notion of community has been adopted as a *political* formation, for it actively challenges the hegemony of dominant ideological constructions of health, identity and lifestyle. But the rhetoric of communities as expressions of political identity and purpose is not a reflection of social reality for drug injectors and their peers. The first step for intervention is to identify communities among drug-injecting networks and next, to create and nurture a shared social responsibility and identity about community health. The associated long-term challenge for networks of drug injectors is to become self-help movements and consumer groups where choices become not merely informed but collectively owned and controlled. While there clearly is a necessity for outreach peer education and community development approaches in this process, it is likely that there will come a point when community organization surpasses the notion of outreach and the need for public health collaboration under so-called *healthy alliances*. It is at this point that intervention among injecting drug users will join an emerging health activism about HIV service provision that will expose the contradictions in the promises and practices of health promotion and the new public health.

Conclusions

Current British models of outreach intervention targeting injecting drug users remain locked into a conception of health promotion which targets individuals and individual behaviour change (Rhodes, 1993). The new public health — and health promotion — advocates the need to balance individual and collective action as a means of enabling changes in individual and collective health status. It advocates the need for community action and community organization in the process of achieving community empowerment and healthy communities. The shift towards a community outreach perspective (ACMD, 1993) attempts to overcome the limits of individualism which continue to plague most UK community-based interventions targeting injecting drug users. The perspective is founded on a health promotion which has an inclusive rather than exclusive understanding of the social bases of health and illness and which locks into the language and the promises of the new public health. It views the community as a target and agent for change. It hopes to facilitate healthy community change by increased community participation and action.

Community action and outreach interventions among injecting drug users remain embryonic. As they emerge, they will have much to learn from the experiences of community action and development within gay communities. In doing so, it is important to ensure that the promises of community outreach are the practices of outreach. This is precisely where the discourse of health promotion and public health performs so well as rhetoric, for there are fundamental contradictions between the promises and practices of the new public health movement. In the light of community action among injecting drug users, these contradictions centre on the potential tensions between the promise of community health and community empowerment and the promise of public health. The promise of public health depends first on what is defined as *health* and second, on what is defined as *public*. It is not clear whether the favoured promise of community empowerment — which is integral to health promotion's much quoted Ottawa Charter — is intended to mean community empowerment in practice. At a preliminary glance, it would appear not. It is going to be increasingly important that community and public health workers stand back from the rhetoric to ponder on the reality. When they do so they should ask: 'Whose side are we on?'.

Acknowledgement

I am grateful to colleagues Gerry Stimson, Alan Quirk and Paul Turnbull for their comments and suggestions on an earlier draft of this chapter.

References

ABDUL-QUADER, A.S., TROSS, S., FRIEDMAN, S.R., KOUZI, A.C. and DES JARLAIS, D.C. (1990) 'Street-recruited intravenous drug users and sexual risk reduction in New York City', *AIDS*, **4**, pp. 1075–79.

ABDUL-QUADER, A.S., TROSS, S., SILVERT, H. *et al.* (1992) 'Peer influence and condom use by female sexual partners of injecting drug users in New York City', Paper presented to VIII International Conference on AIDS, Amsterdam.

ADVISORY COUNCIL ON THE MISUSE OF DRUGS (ACMD) (1988, 1989) *AIDS and Drug Misuse, Parts One and Two*, London: HMSO.

ADVISORY COUNCIL ON THE MISUSE OF DRUGS (ACMD) (1993) *AIDS and Drug Misuse: Update*, London: Department of Health.

AMSEL, Z. (1990) 'Introducing the concept of community prevention', in BATTJES, C.G., AMSEL, D.S.W. and AMSEL, Z. (Eds) *AIDS and Intravenous Drug Use: Future Directions for Community-Based Prevention Research*, Rockville, MD: NIDA Research Monograph 93.

ASHTON, J. and SEYMOUR, H. (1990) *The New Public Health*, Milton Keynes: Open University Press.

BEATTIE, A. (1986) 'Community development for health: From practice to theory', *Radical Health Promotion*, **4**, pp. 12–18.

BEATTIE, A. (1991) 'Knowledge and control in health promotion: A test case for social policy and social theory', in GABE, J., CALNAN, M. and BURY, M. (Eds) *The Sociology of the Health Service*, London: Routledge.

BECKER, H.S. (1963) *Outsiders: Studies in the Sociology of Deviance*, New York: Free Press.

BECKER, H.S. (1967a) 'Whose side are we on?', *Social Problems*, **14**, pp. 239–47.

BECKER, H.S. (1967b) 'History, culture and subjective experience: An exploration of the social bases of drug-induced experiences', *Journal of Health and Social Behaviour*, **8**, pp. 163–76.

BLOOR, M.A., MCKEGANEY, N.P., FINLAY, A. and BARNARD, M.A. (1992) 'The inappropriateness of psycho-social models in explaining the behaviour of rent boys in Glasgow', *AIDS Care*, **4**, pp.1–5.

BROADHEAD, R., HECKATHORN, D.D., GRUND, J.P. and STERN, L.S. (1993) 'Promoting Risk reduction among injecting drug users: A client-driven vs a drug-users union intervention', Paper presented to Fourth International Conference on the Reduction of Drug Related Harm, Rotterdam.

BROWN, E.R. (1991) 'Community action for health promotion: A strategy to empower individuals and communities', *International Journal of Health Services*, **21**, pp. 441–56.

BURROWS, D. and PRICE, C. (1993) 'Peer education among IDUs in Baltimore (US) and Sydney (Australia). Similarities and differences within a model of peer education', Paper presented to IX International Conference on AIDS, Berlin.

BUNTON, R. and MACDONALD, G. (1992) (Eds) *Health Promotion: Disciplines and Diversity*, London: Routledge.

BURT, J. and STIMSON, G.V. (1993) *Injectors and HIV Prevention: Strategies for Protection*, London: Health Education Authority.

CALOUSTE GULBENKIAN FOUNDATION (1984) *A National Centre for Community Development: Report of a Working Party*, London: Gulbenkian Foundation.

CRIMP, D. (Ed.) (1988) *AIDS: Cultural Analysis, Cultural Activism*, London: MIT Press.

DRAPER, P., GRIFFITHS, J., DENNIS, J. and POPAY, J. (1980) 'Three types of health education', *British Medical Journal*, **281**, pp. 493–5.

FARRANT, W. (1991)' Addressing the contradictions: Health promotion and community health action in the United Kingdom', *International Journal of Health Services*, **21**, pp. 423–39.

FRIEDMAN, S.R., DES JARLAIS, D.C., STERK, C. *et al.* (1990) 'AIDS and the social relations of intravenous drug users', *Milbank Quarterly*, 78 (Supp. 1) 85–110.

FRIEDMAN, S.R., JOSE, B., NEAIGUS, A. *et al.* (1991) 'Peer mobilisation and widespread condom use by drug injectors', Paper presented to VIIth International Conference on AIDS, Florence.

FRIEDMAN, S.R., NEAIGUS, A., DES JARLAIS, D.C., SOTHERAN, J.L., WOODS, J., SUFIAN, M., STEPHERSON, and STARK, C. (1992) 'Social intervention against AIDS among injecting drug users', *British Journal of Addiction*, **87**, pp. 393–404.

FRIEDMAN, S.R., DE JONG, W. and WODAK, A. (1993) 'Community development as a response to HIV among drug injectors', *AIDS*, **7** (Supp. 1), S263–9.

GRUND, J.P., BLANKEN, P., ADRIAANS, N.F.P. *et al.* (1992) 'Reaching the unreached: an outreach model for "on the spot" AIDS prevention among active, out of treatment drug addicts,' in O'HARE, P.A. (Ed.) *The Reduction of Drug-Related Harm*, London: Routledge.

HART, G. WOODWARD, N. and CARVELL, A. (1989) 'Needle-exchange in Central London: Operating philosophy and communication strategies', *AIDS Care*, **1**, pp. 125–34.

HENDERSON, P. and THOMAS, D.N. (1980) *Skills in Neighbourhood Work*, London: Allen and Unwin.

HOMANS, H. and AGGLETON, P. (1988) 'Health education about HIV infection and AIDS', in AGGLETON, P. and HOMANS, H. (Eds) *Social Aspects of AIDS*, Lewes: Falmer Press.

HORTON, M. (1989) 'Bugs, drugs and placebos: The opulence of truth, or how to make a treatment decision in an epidemic', in CARTER, E. and WATNEY, S. (Eds) *Taking Liberties: AIDS and Cultural Politics*, London: Serpent's Tail.

KELLY, J.A., ST. LAWRENCE, J.S., DIAZ, Y.E., STEVENSON, L.Y., HAUTH, A.C., BRASFIELD, T.L., KALICHMAN, S.C. (1991) 'HIV-risk behaviour reduction following intervention with key opinion leaders of a population: An experimental community-level analysis', *American Journal of Public Health*, **82**, pp. 168–171.

KELLY, J.A., ST. LAWRENCE, J.S., STEVENSON, L.Y. *et al.* (1992) 'Community AIDS/ HIV risk reduction by enlisting popular people to serve as behaviour change endorsers to their peers: a 3-city sequential replication', *American Journal of Public Health*, **82**, pp. 1482–83.

KIPPAX, S., CRAWFORD, J., CONNELL, B., DOWSETT, G., WATSON, L., RODDEN, P. , BAXTER, D. and RIGMOR, B. (1992) 'The importance of gay community in the prevention of HIV transmission: A study of Australian men who have sex with men', in AGGLETON, P., DAVIES, P. and HART, G. (Eds) *AIDS: Rights, Risk and Reason*, London: Falmer Press.

LABONTE, R. (1989) 'Community empowerment: The need for political analysis', *Canadian Journal of Public Health*, **80**, pp. 87–8.

MACCONNELL D. (1979) 'The elementary structures of community: Macrostructural accounting as a methodology for theory building and policy formation', in BLAKELY, E.J. (Ed.) *Community Development Research*, New York: Human Sciences Press.

MCDERMOTT, P. (1993) 'The personal touch', *Druglink*, **8**, 4, p. 3.

MCKEGANEY, N.P. and BARNARD, M.A. (1992) *AIDS, Drugs and Sexual Risk: Lives in the Balance*, Milton Keynes: Open University Press.

MURPHY, S. (1987) 'Intravenous drug use and AIDS: Notes on the social economy of needle sharing', *Contemporary Drug Problems*, **14**, pp. 272–395.

NATIONAL INSTITUTE OF DRUG ABUSE (NIDA) (1989) *AIDS Outreach in the Community: NIDA Directory of Community Outreach Demonstration Projects and National Resource Organizations*, Rockville, MD: NIDA.

NUTBEAM, D. (1986) 'Health promotion glossary', *Health Promotion*, **1**, pp. 113–27.

NUTBEAM, D. and BLAKEY, V. (1990) 'The concept of health promotion and AIDS prevention: A comprehensive and integrated basis for action in the 1990s', *Health Promotion International*, **5**, pp. 233–42.

O'HARE, P.A., NEWCOMBE, R., MATTHEWS, A., BIRMING, E.C. and DRUCKER, E. (1992) (Eds) *The Reduction of Drug Related Harm*, London: Routledge.

PATTON, C. (1990) *Inventing AIDS*, London: Routledge.

POWER, R., JONES, S., KEANES, G., SMITH, J. and WALD, H. (1993) 'Lifestyles (Part 2): Coping strategies of illicit drug users, final report to the Department of Health', London: Centre for Research on Drugs and Health Behaviour.

RHODES, T.J. and HARTNOLL, R. (1991) 'Reaching the hard to reach: Models of HIV outreach health education', in AGGLETON, P., HART, G. and DAVIES, P. (Eds) *AIDS: Responses, Interventions and Care*, London: Falmer Press.

RHODES, T.J. and HOLLAND, J. (1992) 'Outreach as a strategy for HIV prevention: Aims and practice', *Health Education Research*, 7, pp. 533–46.

RHODES, T.J. (1993) 'Time for community change: What has outreach to offer?', *Addiction*, **88**, pp. 1317–20.

RHODES, T.J. (1994a) *Risk, Intervention and Change: HIV Prevention and Drug Use*, London: Health Education Authority.

RHODES, T.J. (1994b) 'Outreach, peer education and community change', *Health Education Journal* **53**, 1, pp. 92–9.

ROGERS, E.M. and SHOEMAKER, F. (1971) *Communication of Innovations*, New York: Free Press.

ROMER, D. and HORNIK, R. (1992) 'HIV education for youth: The importance of social consensus in behaviour change', *AIDS Care*, **4**, pp. 285–303.

ROSE, H. (1990) 'Activists, gender and the community health movement', *Health Promotion International*, 5, pp. 209–18.

SCHWARTZ, H. and JACOBS, J. (1979) *Qualitative Sociology: A Method to the Madness*, New York: Free Press.

SOTHERAN, J.L., FRIEDMAN, S.R., SUFIAN, M., DES JARLAIS, D.C., ENGEL, S.D., WEBER, J. ROCKWELL, R. and MARMOR, M. (1989) 'Condom use among heterosexual male IV drug users is affected by the nature of social relationships', Paper presented to Vth International Conference on AIDS, Montreal.

STIMSON, G.V. (1990) 'AIDS and HIV: The challenge for British Drugs Services', *British Journal Addiction*, **85**, 3, pp. 329–39.

STIMSON, G.V. (1992) 'Public health and health behaviour in the prevention of HIV infection, in O'HARE, P.A., NEWCOMBE, R., MATTHEWS, A., BURMING, E.C. and DRUCKER, E. (Eds) *The Reduction of Drug Related Harm*, London: Routledge.

STIMSON, G.V. and LART, R. (1991) 'HIV, drugs and public health in England: New words, old tunes', *International Journal of the Addictions*, **26**, pp. 1263–77.

STIMSON, G.V., LART, R., DOLAN, K. and DONOGHOE, M.C. (1991) 'The future of syringe exchange in the public health prevention of HIV infection, in AGGLETON, P., HART, G. and DAVIES, P. (Eds) *AIDS: Responses, Interventions and Care*, London: Falmer Press.

TANNAHILL, A. (1985) 'What is health promotion?', *Health Education Journal*, **44**, pp. 167–8.

THOROGOOD, N. (1992) 'What is the relevance of sociology for health promotion?', in BUNTON, R. and MACDONALD, G. (Eds) *Health Promotion: Disciplines and Diversity*, London: Routledge.

TONES, B.K. (1986) 'Health education and the ideology of health promotion: A review of alternative approaches', *Health Education Research*, **1**, pp. 3–12.

TONES, K., TILFORD, S. and ROBINSON, Y. (1990) *Health Education: Effectiveness and Efficiency*, London: Chapman and Hall.

TROSS, S., ABDUL-QUADER, A.S., SILVERT, H. *et al.* (1992) 'Determinants of condom use in female sexual partners of IV drug users in New York City', Paper presented to the VIIIth International Conference on AIDS, Amsterdam.

WATNEY, S. (1990) 'Safer sex as community practice', in AGGLETON, P., DAVIES, P. and HART, G. (Eds) *AIDS: Individual, Cultural and Policy Dimensions*, London: Falmer Press.

Tim Rhodes

WIEBEL, W. (1988) 'Combining ethnographic and epidemiological methods in targeted AIDS interventions: The Chicago model', in BATTJES, R. and PICKENS, R. (Eds) *Needle Sharing Among Intravenous Drug Abusers: National and International Perspectives*, Rockville, MD: NIDA Monograph 80.

WORLD HEALTH ORGANIZATION AND CANADIAN PUBLIC HEALTH ASSOCIATION (1986) 'Ottawa Charter for Health Promotion', *Health Promotion*, **1**, pp. iii–v.

Chapter 5

Project Male-call: Class Differences in Sexual Practice

Pam Rodden, June Crawford and Susan Kippax

In mid-1992, the National Centre for HIV Social Research conducted a telephone survey of homosexual practice, *Project Male-Call* (Kippax, Crawford and Rodden, 1993), as part of an evaluation of the Australian Government's HIV/AIDS strategy. The survey focused on men who have sex with men and was designed to collect data relevant to HIV/AIDS prevention, particularly information concerning sexual practices and knowledge about HIV/AIDS.

In 1986/7 a similar Australian study, the Social Aspects of the Prevention of AIDS (SAPA), had surveyed men from New South Wales (Kippax, Connell, Dowsett and Crawford, 1993). The men in this study, who were recruited in the main from Sydney, the capital of New South Wales, were better educated and more affluent than the general population (Connell, Crawford, Kippax *et al.*, 1988), and to a very large extent, attached to a gay community (Kippax, Crawford, Connell, *et al.*, 1992). In the hope of extending and complementing the findings of previous research, recruitment for *Project Male-Call* targeted men who lived outside the gay areas of Sydney and Melbourne, the other city in Australia with a large gay population. It also targeted men who had little connection with usual avenues of gay social contact, as well as those who were gay community attached. It aimed to reach a higher proportion of working class men and a higher proportion of men from non English-speaking backgrounds.

There are very few studies which have examined the influence of class on homosexual practice. Reiche and Danneker (1977) suggested that male homosexual *identity* might promote social mobility and lead to class advantage, and found some evidence for this in terms of educational achievement. In their study they also noted a preference for white-collar over blue-collar occupations. On the other hand, Kinsey, Pomeroy and Martin (1948) found a substantial level of homosexual practice among manual workers, while Schofield (1965) in a British study of sexual practice of youth found little difference between social classes. There are also very few studies examining class as a factor associated with HIV transmission, either among homosexual or heterosexual populations. Given that studies carried out in the developing world often cite poverty and social disruption as factors associated with increased risk of HIV transmission, this comparative absence is odd.

The studies which have examined the adoption of safe sex among homosexually active men indicate that those who are socially and economically disadvantaged are less likely to have adopted safe sexual practices as a response to HIV/AIDS. In Australia, early research in New South Wales hinted at important class differences in sexual practice (Connell, Dowsett, Rodden and Davis, 1991). There were significant associations between class, defined by educational level achieved, occupational and labour force status, and income, on the one hand, and sexual practice, on the other. In relation to expression of sexuality, working-class men were found to engage in slightly fewer oral/tactile practices and more unprotected anal sex with occasional or casual partners. In comparison with other homosexually active men, they were also more likely to enjoy sex with women. Men with lower incomes were less likely to use condoms, and receptive anal intercourse with casual partners was more likely among those with least education and those in a wage-labour economic position. The analyses showed that the relationships between measures of social class and sexual practice were, in the main, independent of attachment to gay community. There were, indeed, few class differences with regard to measures of attachment to gay community, although working class men were less likely to belong to gay organizations than men from the middle or upper classes (Dowsett, Davis and Connell, 1992).

Similar findings were reported from two studies undertaken outside Australia. In a study examining the correlates of unsafe sexual practice in three sites in the United States, Doll, Byers, Bolan, *et al.* (1991) identified men with low incomes and high levels of sexual activity as one of two groups of men who engaged in most high-risk anal intercourse. In the Netherlands, deWit, van Griensven, Kok and Sandfort (1993) identified a number of variables which were significantly correlated with a return to unprotected anal intercourse with casual partners. One of the correlates was employment status: 81.5 per cent of the men who had maintained protected anal intercourse with casual partners were employed, while only 63.8 per cent of the unemployed men had done so.

Several speakers at the IXth International Conference on AIDS in Berlin, notably Rosenbrock (1993) and Bassett (1993), reviewed literature that indicated the negative impact of social and economic disadvantage on people's ability to prevent HIV transmission. Three studies each examining the impact of class on sexual practice in a different population report similar results. In a study of 3601 male and female clients of the main HIV counselling and testing clinic in Seattle, Washington, in the United States, Krueger, Wood, Diehr and Maxwell (1990) found that self-reported income level was related to HIV seropositivity; the authors noting that this effect was independent of race and age. Osmond, Wambach, Byers, Levine, and Quadagno (1993) who surveyed a sample of over

690 women in Florida found similar results: the effects of class, as measured by years of education and source of income, and race were multiplicative. In a study of injecting drug users, Brown, Chu, Nemoto, *et al.* (1989) found that injecting drug users who had comparatively more years of education and legitimate employment had lower rates of HIV infection. There is no reason to believe that homosexually active men are any different in this regard. The purpose of this chapter is to re-examine the relationship between knowledge of HIV transmission, sexual practice, both safe and unsafe, HIV infection rates and social class.

Method

The findings discussed here come from a national telephone survey of 2583 homosexually active men conducted in the middle of 1992 in Australia.

Questionnaire

The questionnaire, which was based on the earlier SAPA questionnaire, covered knowledge of HIV transmission, sexual practice with men and women, and included a wide range of demographic and milieu or context variables. The questionnaire took, on average, about 45 minutes to administer.

For inclusion in the survey, respondents were required to have had 'sex with a man' during the five years prior to the survey. Men were recruited via AIDS Councils, video mailing lists, personal advertisements in local newspapers, radio interviews, fliers and posters in bars, saunas and discos. They were asked to ring on a toll free number any day between the hours of 10 am and 10 pm. The lines were open from 1 May to 30 June. Trained interviewers, both men and women, took the calls and administered the questionnaire.

Just under 7500 telephone calls were recorded. There were 2667 completed interviews and 257 incomplete interviews. Of the completed interviews, a number contained gross errors or inconsistencies and were excluded from analysis. The final sample was 2583 men. The remainder of the 7491 calls were received at times when there were either insufficient interviewers on duty or insufficient telephone lines available. Respondents who were willing to leave a telephone number were called back, or they themselves called back. We estimate (and stress that this is based on very incomplete data) that we interviewed 50 per cent of those whose calls were recorded. There would have been a further number of men who, because of busy lines, never reached us.

Sample characteristics

There is no way of knowing whether the sample achieved is representative of homosexually active men in Australia. The sample as a whole, however, comprised men from all states of Australia. While there was a slight under-representation of men from Western Australia, the spread was otherwise good. In comparison with the 1991 Australian Census data, and in common with other studies of gay men (Davies, 1986), there was an over-representation of tertiary educated and professional men in this sample, and an under-representation of men under 18 and over 50 years. Atheists and agnostics were also over-represented. Men were predominantly from anglo-celtic backgrounds, and the sample under-represented men from non English-speaking backgrounds.

The sample of men was, however, a heterogeneous one and it differs from samples in earlier studies in Australia (Tindall, Swanson, Donovan and Cooper, 1989; Kippax, Connell, Dowsett and Crawford, 1993) in the larger proportion of men identifying as heterosexual (3.7 per cent) or bisexual (26.9 per cent), and men sexually interested in women (only 60.1% reported enjoying sex with 'men only').

Almost three quarters of the sample had a social attachment to gay community while one quarter of the men had few gay male friends and spent little time with gay male friends. Just over 74 per cent of the sample had been antibody tested and 9 per cent of those tested were seropositive. Only 32 per cent knew no one who had HIV or AIDS, while over half (52.9 per cent) knew someone who had died of AIDS, and 26 per cent had cared for someone with AIDS.

Measures of Class

Three indicators of class were considered since there is no single best measure (Connell, Dowsett, Rodden and Davis, 1991). In the context of this study, class is considered to be a loose construct, related to education and occupation. As other studies, for example Doll, Byers, Bolan *et al.* (1991), used income as an index of class this factor is also included, being often associated with educational level and occupation. Other variables included in the study that may also be class-related are self attributed sexual identity, gay community attachment and place of residence. The three class variables were as follows:

- *Education* was defined in four groups:
    i) those with education up to Year 10, called the Lower Secondary group;
    ii) those with Senior Secondary education;
    iii) those with tertiary diplomas or trade certificates, called the Post Secondary group;

iv) and those with Higher Education, at the level of undergraduate or postgraduate study.

- *Occupation* was defined in terms of five categories:
  - i) manager/professional;
  - ii) paraprofessional/clerical;
  - iii) sales/service;
  - iv) trade/manual;
  - v) no job, a mixed group which includes students, those out of the workforce, those on social security and the unemployed.

- *Income* was defined in terms of four groups of annual income:
  - i) less than $15 000;
  - ii) $15 001–$26 000;
  - iii) $26 001–$40 000;
  - iv) more than $40 000.

As might be expected, there were highly significant statistical associations ($p \approx 0.0000$ for all three tests of association) between the three measures. On examination of the relationships between each of the three indicators of class and context and outcome variables, education and occupation gave similar results. Few variables differed along income lines. For the sake of simplicity, therefore, we use occupation as the major indicator of class in the remainder of this chapter.

Results

The focus of this chapter was to determine whether sexual practice, HIV knowledge and the adoption of safe sex differ significantly according to class, and in particular whether class differences in these variables are merely a reflection of other demographic or contextual (milieu) variables. A number of univariate analyses investigated class differences with regard to a range of variables, under four general headings: demographic variables (including sexual identity); milieu or context variables; knowledge of HIV; and safe and unsafe sexual practice. The results are discussed using occupation as a marker of class. Reference will be made to education and income differences only if such data add to the understanding of the results. Multivariate analyses of covariance were also carried out to test the hypothesis that over and above milieu and demographic variables, class is an important explanatory variable of HIV knowledge and sexual practice, both safe and unsafe.

Univariate Analyses

Demographic variables

Significant relationships were found between occupation and several important demographic variables. These included age, place of residence, marital status and living arrangements. No significant relationship was found with country of birth. With respect to age, few men in managerial/professional jobs were under 25, while a high proportion of those with no job were under 25. A relatively low proportion of those aged between 25 and 40 had no job ($p \approx 0.0000$). Men in trade/manual occupations were more likely to live in rural areas and non-gay urban areas ($p \approx 0.0000$), to have been married ($p \approx 0.0000$), and to live with a female partner and/or children ($p \approx 0.0000$).

There were also differences between the men with regard to sexual identity and sexual preference. In particular, those in trade/manual occupations were more likely to self identify as bisexual or heterosexual (52.6 per cent) than those in other occupation categories (which were very similar, varying from 24 per cent to 28 per cent) ($p \approx 0.0000$). Men in trade/manual occupations were also more likely to report that they enjoyed having sex with men and women: 44.6 per cent said that they enjoyed sex with 'men and women' or 'mostly women' or 'women only', compared with around 20 per cent in the other occupation groups ($p \approx 0.0000$).

Milieu variables

Men in the different occupational categories also differed significantly on a number of milieu variables. An important group of milieu variables were gay community attachment, contact with the HIV epidemic, and disclosure of gay identity. Scales were formed to measure three aspects of attachment to gay community. The three gay community attachment scales were social engagement, cultural/political involvement and sexual engagement, being similar to those which we used in previous research (Kippax *et al.*, 1992). Two other scales, which measured degree of contact with the epidemic and disclosure of homosexual activity, were also formed. Significant occupation differences were found on all of these scales, as shown in Table 5.1.

The statistical tests used were one-way analyses of variance to test the significance of the differences among the means. In each case, the trade/manual occupation category was significantly different from the remainder, with the exception of the Sexual Engagement Scale where the mean for the group with no job was similar to that for the trade/manual category. The trade/manual group had low levels of attachment to gay community, contact with the epidemic, and disclosure of gay identity.

Table 5.1   Means and standard deviations of gay community attachment and milieu scales

	Manager/ Professional n = 928	Paraprof/ Clerical n = 414	Trade/ Manual n = 424	Sales/ Service n = 303	No Job n = 501
Social Engagement***					
Mean	7.8	7.7	5.8	7.7	7.3
SD	3.5	3.5	3.6	3.8	3.6
Gay Involvement***					
Mean	2.0	1.9	1.4	1.9	1.9
SD	1.0	1.0	1.0	1.0	1.0
Contact with Epidemic***					
Mean	1.6	1.4	0.8	1.3	1.3
SD	1.1	1.1	1.0	1.1	1.1
Sexual Engagement**					
	n = 905	n = 402	n = 408	n = 293	n = 489
Mean	20.4	20.2	19.7	20.3	19.7
SD	3.9	3.8	3.8	4.3	3.8
Disclosure of Gay Identity***					
	n = 848	n = 394	n = 404	n = 272	n = 450
Mean	3.2	3.1	1.8	3.0	2.9
SD	2.2	2.2	2.0	2.3	2.3

*** $p \approx 0.0000$
** $p < 0.01$

Table 5.2   Test status: Per cent of men

	Manager/ Professional n = 928	Paraprof/ Clerical n = 414	Trade/ Manual n = 424	Sales/ Service n = 303	No Job n = 501
Test Status***					
No Test/Result	21.3	20.5	37.5	22.1	28.5
HIV Positive	6.5	6.3	3.1	6.9	10.2
HIV Negative	72.2	73.2	59.4	71.0	61.3

*** $p \approx 0.0000$

There was also a significant relationship ($p \approx 0.0000$) between HIV/AIDS test status and occupation (see Table 5.2). Men in trade/manual occupations were significantly less likely to have been tested, and among those who had been tested, those with no occupation were significantly more likely to be HIV positive than those who were employed ($p < 0.0001$).

Table 5.3   *Means and standard deviations of knowledge scales*

	Manager/ Professional n = 928	Paraprof/ Clerical n = 414	Trade/ Manual n = 424	Sales/ Service n = 303	No Job n = 501
SCALE					
Transmission of Virus***					
Mean	5.71	5.65	5.51	5.66	5.67
SD	0.57	0.61	0.71	0.57	0.62
KnowunsafeM***					
Mean	1.77	1.72	1.61	1.69	1.65
SD	0.44	0.48	0.55	0.48	0.54
KnowunsafeW*					
Mean	3.31	3.26	3.11	3.26	3.27
SD	0.97	1.02	1.17	0.98	1.07

* $p < 0.05$
** $p < 0.01$
*** $p < 0.001$

Accuracy of Knowledge

A number of scales measured accuracy of knowledge about HIV and the safety of sexual practices. Overall the level of knowledge within the sample was high, with only small occupational group differences in the means. Some differences were, however, statistically significant.

There were differences for knowledge of transmission of the virus, the Transmission Scale; of unsafe unprotected anal intercourse with men, the KnowunsafeM Scale; and to a lesser extent, of unsafe unprotected anal and vaginal intercourse with women, the KnowunsafeW Scale. In all cases, those working in trade/ manual occupations had the least accurate knowledge (see Table 5.3). The knowledge scales for which there were no occupation–related differences were knowledge of the effectiveness of condoms in sex with men and in sex with women, KnowsafeM and KnowsafeW Scales.

Sexual practice variables

With respect to their current relationship status with men (Table 5.4), those employed in trade/manual occupations were more likely than other occupational groups to have casual sex only. Those in professional or sales/service occupations were the most likely to have some form of regular relationship.

Compared with other occupational groups, trade/manual workers had had fewer male sexual partners in the six months prior to the survey ($p < 0.003$) and over a lifetime ($p \approx 0.0000$). The professional men and those earning more than \$40 000 ($p < 0.006$) had had the most male partners. With respect to sex with

Table 5.4   Relationship status: Per cent of men in each category

	Manager/ Professional n = 928	Paraprof/ Clerical n = 414	Trade/ Manual n = 424	Sales/ Service n = 303	No Job n = 501
Relationship Status**					
None	7.4	9.0	11.1	4.3	11.0
Monogamous	17.8	19.9	15.1	21.8	21.2
Regular plus casual	23.7	19.1	15.6	20.1	15.2
Several regular	3.3	3.6	4.7	4.3	3.8
Casual Only	47.5	48.4	53.3	49.5	48.9
Other	0.2	0.0	0.2	0.0	0.0

** p $<$ 0.01

women, in both the previous six months and ever, trade/manual workers and those in the highest income group had had the most female sexual partners (p $\approx$ 0.000 and p $\approx$ 0.000 for occupation; p $<$ 0.004 and p $\approx$ 0.000 for income).

When sexual repertoire was examined, there were once again many differences with respect to occupation. The sexual repertoire of the men was analysed by examining both the frequency with which men engaged in particular activities and the range of sexual behaviours in which they engaged. The range was assessed in terms of four scales: the Anal scale, which consisted of eight items (insertive and receptive forms of anal intercourse with and without ejaculation, rimming, and fingering); the Soft scale which was made up of six items (wet/deep and dry kissing, insertive and receptive oral-genital sex without semen swallowed or ejaculated, mutual masturbation, and sensuous touching); the Swallow/ejaculate scale, which consisted of two items (insertive and receptive oral-genital sex with semen swallowed or ejaculated into partner's mouth); and the Fisting scale which consisted of two items (fisting and being fisted). High scores on these scales indicated a larger repertoire of practice.

Those working in trade/manual occupations were the distinctive group with regard to both frequency and range of sexual behaviours. Men in trade/ manual occupations engaged in fewer oral/tactile practices with men as measured on the Soft scale (p $<$ 0.0005), and engaged in these practices less frequently, particularly with casual partners (Tables 5.5 & 5.6). These same men were, however, more likely than other occupational groups to swallow semen and/or ejaculate into their partner's mouth during oral sex and to engage in more of these practices as measured on the Swallow/Ejaculate scale (p $<$ 0.0005), and, although few men engaged in the practice, men in trade/manual occupations and men from sales and service occupations engaged in more fisting (p $<$ 0.005) as measured by the Fisting scale.

No occupation-related differences were found with regard to the Anal scale. There were no occupation–related differences in the frequency of anal sex (Table

Table 5.5 Sexual practices ('often' or 'occasionally') with regular partner/s in last six months: Per cent of men engaging in each practice

	Manager/ Professional n = 435	Paraprof/ Clerical n = 181	Trade/ Manual n = 155	Sales/ Service n = 146	No Job n = 210
SEXUAL PRACTICE					
Sensuous touching	99.1	99.4	97.4	98.6	97.6
Deep kissing*	93.8	96.1	87.0	91.8	90.5
Dry Kissing	92.6	94.4	87.7	91.1	91.9
Mutual masturbation	94.2	96.1	96.7	92.5	93.8
Oral-genital (no ejaculation)					
-giving	92.4	92.2	90.3	91.1	91.9
-receiving	87.3	89.9	86.4	85.6	87.6
Oral-genital (with ejaculation)					
-giving	38.0	40.0	44.2	36.3	41.9
-receiving*	40.4	43.3	56.5	39.7	44.8
Anal fingering					
-giving	67.5	68.9	71.4	69.9	65.7
-receiving	64.7	67.2	66.9	71.9	60.0
Anal intercourse					
-insertive	56.9	53.0	62.6	59.6	54.3
-receptive	56.4	49.2	59.4	55.5	55.2
Anal with withdrawal					
-insertive	36.3	31.1	40.6	42.5	33.8
-receptive	35.8	33.1	38.7	35.6	33.3
Rimming					
-giving	47.5	51.7	51.9	51.4	48.6
-receiving	49.1	58.3	58.4	56.2	51.0
Fisting					
-giving*	5.5	7.8	11.7	12.3	6.2
-receiving**	5.5	8.9	12.3	14.4	6.7

* $p < 0.05$
** $p < 0.01$
*** $p < 0.001$

5.5) or condom use with regular male partners. When sex with casual male partners was examined, however, those employed in trade/manual occupations were likely to engage in receptive anal sex more frequently (Table 5.6) and less likely to use condoms, or to use them inconsistently (Table 5.7). The same group of men were also less likely to use lubricants with condoms ($p \approx 0.0000$) and when they did, were more likely to use oil based ones ($p < 0.0001$).

The above findings of the univariate analyses indicate that men in trade/manual occupations stand out from men in other occupational categories. These men, too, are the least well educated. To summarize: in general, men in trade/manual occupations were less likely to identify as gay, disclose their homosexual activity, live in urban gay areas, live alone or with other men in a regular

Table 5.6   Sexual practices ('often' or 'occasionally') with casual partner/s in the last six months: Per cent of men engaging in each practice

	Manager/ Professional n = 703	Paraprof/ Clerical n = 303	Trade/ Manual n = 308	Sales/ Service n = 217	No Job n = 350
SEXUAL PRACTICE					
Sensuous touching**	97.3	97.4	92.4	97.7	94.9
Deep kissing***	80.6	85.8	67.8	77.4	81.4
Dry Kissing***	80.9	87.1	66.8	76.5	78.3
Mutual masturbation**	95.4	95.0	88.8	92.6	92.0
Oral-genital (no ejaculation)					
-giving***	90.0	91.1	81.3	84.8	88.0
-receiving**	90.3	87.5	82.2	86.6	85.1
Oral-genital (with ejaculation)					
-giving***	21.0	22.1	36.0	21.7	27.7
-receiving***	36.9	34.7	56.8	40.1	43.0
Anal fingering					
-giving	59.9	61.4	58.4	65.4	57.1
-receiving	57.1	60.7	59.0	66.8	60.6
Anal intercourse					
-insertive	40.5	42.6	48.7	44.7	40.6
-receptive***	31.9	36.0	45.9	35.3	38.9
Anal with withdrawal					
-insertive	26.4	27.4	25.7	29.4	24.8
-receptive	22.3	24.4	27.1	23.4	26.0
Rimming					
-giving	32.9	38.0	38.9	39.2	34.9
-receiving*	45.5	50.8	53.6	55.8	49.1
Fisting					
-giving	7.6	8.3	12.8	8.8	9.1
-receiving***	4.9	6.9	12.5	6.9	7.1

* $p < 0.05$
** $p < 0.01$
*** $p < 0.001$

relationship, and have an exclusive sexual preference for men. They were also less likely to be attached to gay community, and to have been tested for HIV. They were, on the other hand, more likely to have sex with women and to have had more female and fewer male partners than men in other occupational groups. These same men were likely to have engaged in more oral-genital sex with semen exchange, either ejaculating or swallowing semen. Men in trade/ manual occupations were also more likely than men in other occupational groups to engage in anal sexual practices without condoms with casual partners; practices which are considered unsafe. Men in the trade/manual occupations were also those who had the least accurate knowledge of HIV transmission and risk practices.

Table 5.7   *Condom use in anal sex with casual partner/s in the last six months: Per cent of men*

	Manager/ Professional n = 703	Paraprof/ Clerical n = 303	Trade/ Manual n = 308	Sales/ Service n = 217	No Job n = 350
SEXUAL PRACTICE					
Insertive anal**	n = 284	n = 130	n = 150	n = 98	n = 144
Never	7.0	7.7	15.3	3.1	9.0
Sometimes	10.6	4.6	14.7	12.2	15.3
Always	82.4	87.7	70.0	84.7	75.7
Receptive anal	n = 224	n = 109	n = 141	n = 77	n = 136
Never	8.0	5.5	12.1	5.2	8.1
Sometimes	8.5	8.3	16.3	10.4	9.6
Always	83.5	86.2	71.6	84.4	82.4
Insertive anal with withdrawal**					
	n = 186	n = 83	n = 80	n = 64	n = 89
Never	15.1	8.4	25.0	9.4	7.9
Sometimes	10.8	21.7	16.3	7.8	19.1
Always	74.2	69.9	58.8	82.8	73.0
Receptive anal with withdrawal*					
	n = 157	n = 75	n = 83	n = 51	n = 93
Never	11.5	9.3	16.9	9.8	6.5
Sometimes	10.8	13.3	21.7	3.9	14.0
Always	77.7	77.3	61.4	86.3	79.6

* $p < 0.05$
** $p < 0.01$
*** $p < 0.001$

Multivariate class analyses

The simple comparisons outlined above raise several questions about the complex inter-relationship of influences. We know from previous research (e.g. Kippax *et al.*, 1993) that differences in knowledge and especially in attachment to gay community are important in influencing sexual practice and behaviour change.

A series of multivariate analyses of covariance and logistic regressions were carried out in order to investigate whether the impact of class on knowledge and sexual practice could be explained by class differences in demographic variables (age, income, and place of residence (region)) and/or in gay community attachment and other milieu variables. Place of residence (region) was included as a design variable, and since region was correlated with both education and occupation, the analyses were done with region fitted first in order to examine the effect of occupation or education when adjusted for region. The covariates in all analyses were: age, income, self-attributed sexual identity, relationship status, number of male sexual partners ever, whether sex with women was enjoyed, the three gay community attachment scales, and contact with the epidemic.

The three groups of variables of interest were: HIV knowledge, as measured by the five knowledge scales, Knowledge of Transmission (Knowtransm), KnowsafeM, KnowsafeW, KnowunsafeM, and KnowunsafeW; sexual practice, as measured by the four sexual practice scales, Anal, Soft, Swallow/Ejaculate and Fisting scales; and safe/unsafe sex as measured in terms of whether or not anal sex with a casual partner was with or without a condom (SafCas).

Separate analyses were carried out examining education differences and occupation differences with regard to each of the three groups described above. There were thus six analyses in all. The multivariate tests of the effect of education on knowledge and sexual practice were significant, $p \approx 0.000$ and $p \approx 0.000$, respectively. The multivariate test of the effect of occupation on knowledge was not significant, although the multivariate test of the effect of occupation on sexual practice was significant, $p \approx 0.000$. The effect of education and — separately — of occupation on safety of anal sex with casual partners was assessed using logistic regression analyses. These two analyses were based on the 1158 men who had anal sex with their casual partners. Education was statistically significantly related to safety of anal sex with casual partners; the greater the number of years of education, the more likely that condoms were used. There was no effect for occupation. The results of the univariate tests of significance, taking all covariates and region into account, are summarized in Table 5.8.

Occupation differences in HIV knowledge were found to be accounted for by demographic and milieu variables. Education differences in HIV knowledge, however, remained significant after adjustment for demographic and milieu variables ($p \approx 0.000$). These results confirmed that the relationship between education and knowledge of unsafe sexual practices referred to in the section on univariate results above were not merely a reflection of differences in gay community attachment, for example.

Both education and occupation differences remained significant with respect to sexual practice as assessed on the sexual practice scales. There were significant effects on oral-genital sex with semen exchange (Swal/Ejac) and also on soft practices such as masturbation, kissing, and sensuous touching. Men in trade/manual occupations and with lower educational achievement engaged in a smaller range of soft practices but more oral-genital practices with swallowing and/or ejaculation. Fisting was found to vary significantly with education but not with occupation; men with higher levels of education engaged in fewer fisting practices. Although there was not a significant effect of occupation on condom use for anal intercourse with casual partners, there was a significant effect of education. Men with low levels of education were less likely to use condoms in anal intercourse with casual partners.

The outcome of the multivariate and logistic regression analyses confirms that class (as indicated by education and occupational status) has an impact on sexual practice. This relationship between occupation and sexual practice is not

Table 5.8 *Summary of results of univariate analyses for three sets of variables examining 'class'*

Effect after covariate adjustment	F	d.f.	p
Knowledge Scales — Region × Education			
Knowtransm	12.37	3,2299	.000
KnowsafeM	2.63	3,2299	.049
KnowsafeW	4.80	3,2299	.002
KnowunsafeM	3.21	3,2299	.022
KnowunsafeW	4.77	3,2299	.003
Knowledge Scales — Region × Occupation			
Knowtransm	2.19	4,2287	.068
KnowsafeM	0.68	4,2287	.603
KnowsafeW	0.34	4,2287	.848
KnowunsafeM	2.90	4,2287	.021
KnowunsafeW	0.23	4,2287	.920
Sexual Practices Scales: Region × Education			
Anal	1.11	3,2293	.343
Soft	3.56	3,2293	.014
Swal/ejac	5.64	3,2293	.001
Fisting	6.33	3,2293	.000
Sexual Practices Scales: Region × Occupation			
Anal	1.03	4,2281	.391
Soft	3.50	4,2281	.007
Swal/ejac	4.98	4,2281	.001
Fisting	1.95	4,2281	.187
Anal Sex with Casual Partners:			
Education: Chi Square 13.55 with 3 d.f, p = 0.004			
Occupation: Chi Square 3.97 with 4 d.f. p = 0.411			

a reflection of gay community attachment, contact with the epidemic, sexual identity, enjoying sex with women, place of residence, age, or income, but appears to be a direct effect of class. It is important to note, however, that although there is evidence for social disadvantage to be related to unsafe sexual practice with casual partners, the evidence relates to years of education and, to a lesser degree, to trade/manual occupational status. The relationship between class and HIV seropositivity, on the other hand, is not based on educational achievement but is tied to lack of employment.

Discussion

To summarize the findings of the class analysis: in comparison with other men, men in trade/manual occupations, working class men, were more likely to self-identify as heterosexual or bisexual and to enjoy sex with women. They were far less involved in gay community, knew less about HIV/AIDS and unsafe sexual practices, were less likely to have been tested for HIV, had a different pattern of sexual practice with men, and were more likely to engage in unsafe anal practices with casual partners. Findings which were hinted at in the earlier SAPA study (Connell, Dowsett, Rodden and Davis, 1991) were highly significant in the analysis of Male-Call data, probably because Male-Call recruitment strategies were successful in their attempt to reach men outside gay community.

Class differences in knowledge show that working class men are disadvantaged with regard to some information about HIV/AIDS. Gay community based programs are unlikely to reach them. Even those working class men who are attached to gay community engage in a restricted range of the safe 'soft' practices while continuing with other sexual behaviour which places them and their partners at risk.

The data reported here indicate that not only are working-class men and men with lower levels of education more likely to engage in unsafe sexual practices, but the form of their sexual practice differs. These findings indicate, as do the findings of Kinsey, Pomeroy and Martin (1948), that working class men engage in homosexual activity, but they do not support Schofield's (1965) findings of few class differences in sexual activity. It is, however, notable that the differences in sexual activity, especially when viewed alongside the differences with regard to self-attributed identity, sexual interest in women, and predominance of casual only relations with men, suggest that 'gayness' may be a middle class concept, as Reiche and Danneker (1977) propose, and that male-to-male sex is constructed differently for working-class men.

In more general terms, the findings demonstrate that it is important to distinguish sexual practice itself, the sexual repertoire, from changes in sexual practice as a response to the HIV/AIDS epidemic. With regard to unsafe practices, the results reported here confirm findings from the Netherlands (deWit *et al.*, 1993); education is implicated in the up-take of safe sexual practices. It is important to note, however, that the men who took part in Male-Call could not be called poor. There was a range across occupational and educational status, but the poverty and social disruption reported by Rosenbrock (1993) and Bassett (1993) is most likely very different for the men in this study. HIV transmission in Australia has occurred predominantly among gay rather than homosexually–active men. Such self-identified gay men are more likely to be well educated and to have middle class occupations. Among the sample of men in this study, there is, however, evidence of a relationship between unemployment, a form of social and economic disadvantage, and HIV seropositivity. It is possible that unemployment is an effect of HIV infection rather than its cause.

References

BASSETT, M.T. (1993) 'Social and economic determinants of vulnerability to HIV', Plenary presentation at the *IXth International Conference on AIDS*, Berlin.

BROWN, L.S., CHU, A., NEMOTO, T. AJULUCHUKWU, D., PRIMM, B.J. (1989) 'Human immunodeficiency virus infection in a cohort of intravenous drug users in New York City: Demographic, behavioural and clinical features', *New York State Journal of Medicine*, **89**, 9, pp. 506–10.

CONNELL, R.W., CRAWFORD, J., KIPPAX, S., DOWSETT, G.W., BOND, G., BAXTER,D., BERG, R. and WATSON, L. (1988) 'Method and sample: Social Aspects of the Prevention of AIDS, Study A, Report No. 1', Sydney: Macquarie University.

CONNELL, R.W., DOWSETT, G.W., RODDEN, P. and DAVIS, M.D. (1991) 'Social class, gay men and AIDS prevention', *Australian Journal of Public Health*, **15**, 3, pp. 178–89.

DAVIES, P.M. (1986) 'Some problems in defining and sampling non-heterosexual males', Project Sigma Working Paper No 3. Cardiff: University of Cardiff, Department of Sociology.

DEWIT, J.B.F., VAN GRIENSVEN, G.J.P., KOK, G. and SANDFORT, T.G.M. (1993) 'Why do homosexual men relapse into unsafe sex? Predictors of resumption of unprotected anogenital intercourse with casual partners', *AIDS*, 7, pp. 1113–18.

DOLL. L.S., BYERS R.H., BOLAN, G., DOUGLAS, J.M., MOSS, P.M., WELLER, P.D., JOY, D., BARTHOLOW, B.N. and HARRISON, J.S. (1991) 'Homosexual men who engage in high-risk sexual behaviour: A multicenter comparison', *Sexually Transmitted Diseases*, **18**, pp. 170–5.

DOWSETT, G.W., DAVIS, M.D. and CONNELL, R.W. (1992) 'Working-class homosexuality and HIV/AIDS prevention: Some recent research from Sydney, Australia', *Psychology and Health*, **6**, pp. 313–24.

KINSEY, A.C., POMEROY, W.D. and MARTIN, C.E. (1948) *Sexual Behaviour in the Human Male*, Philadelphia, PA: WB Saunders.

KIPPAX, S., CONNELL, R.W., DOWSETT, G.W. and CRAWFORD, J. (1993) *Sustaining Safe Sex: Gay Communities Respond to AIDS*, London: Falmer Press.

KIPPAX, S., CRAWFORD, J., CONNELL, R.W., DOWSETT, G,, WATSON L., RODDEN, P., BAXTER, D. and BERG, R. (1992). 'The importance of gay community in the prevention of HIV transmission: A study of Australian men who have sex with men', in AGGLETON, P., DAVIES, P. and HART G. (Eds). *AIDS, Rights, Risk and Reason*, London: Falmer Press.

KIPPAX, S., CRAWFORD, J. and RODDEN, P. (1993) *Project Male-Call: A National Telephone Survey of Homosexually Active Men: A Report to the Commonwealth Department of Health, Housing and Community Services*, Canberra.

KRUEGER, L.E., WOOD, R.W., DIEHR, P.H. and MAXWELL, C.L. (1990) 'Poverty and HIV seropositivity: the poor are more likely to be infected', *AIDS*, **4**, pp. 811–14.

OSMOND, M.W., WAMBACH, K.G., HARRISON, D.F., BYERS, J., LEVINE, P., IMERSHEIN, A. and QUADAGNO, D.M. (1993) 'The multiple jeopardy of race, class, and gender for AIDS risk among Women', *Gender and Society*, 7, 1, pp. 99–120.

REICHE R. and DANNEKER, M. (1977) 'Male homosexuality in West Germany — a sociological investigation', *Journal of Sex Research*, **13**, 1, pp. 35–53.

ROSENBROCK, R. (1993) 'The role of policy in effective prevention: education and care, plenary presentation at the *IXth International Conference on AIDS*, Berlin.

SCHOFIELD, M. (1965) *The Sexual Behaviour of Young People*, London: Longmans.

TINDALL, B., SWANSON, C., DONOVAN, B. and COOPER, D.A. (1989) 'Sexual practices and condom usage in a cohort of homosexual men in relation to human immunodeficiency virus status', *Medical Journal of Australia*, **151**, pp. 318–22.

Chapter 6

Community vs. Population: The Case of Men who have Sex with Men

Michael Bartos

Of the various ways of understanding HIV/AIDS, I want to focus on its connection to government. In part, this means looking at HIV/AIDS policies. But one problem with much policy analysis is that it tends to regard as a given the problem in response to which any particular policy is developed. In this chapter I hope to uncover more of the conditions of possibility for the framing of HIV/AIDS policies, and that means casting the net of government widely. Small 'g' government is sometimes conflated with big 'G' Government. The public sector and Government budgets are taken to cover the field of government. There is, however, another usage of government which encompasses the full array of institutions and administrative practices under which social life is governed. For example, Simey, in his 1937 book *Principles of Social Administration*, included the following services in government:

> 'Personal' Health Services; Public Assistance; Education; House Property Management; Unemployment Relief . . . and Vocational Guidance; National Health Insurance; Pensions; Lunacy and Mental Deficiency; Home Office 'Reformative Services' including the Prisons.
> (Simey, 1937:6)

together with

> the services which have since been called 'environmental', such as street-cleansing, refuse-disposal, drainage and water supply. Services of this type seek to improve the sanitary (or generally speaking, the physical) surroundings of the individual, and thus indirectly lead to public health, or greater amenities of life.
> (Simey, 1937:4)

Whether in Simey's list, or in an updated version, all these amenities and functions are subject to administration. They have developed particular administrative technologies and knowledge. They constitute in particular ways the subject on which they act, whether as a customer, a consumer, a citizen or an inmate. In this respect, Nikolas Rose has suggested,

> Government, in the sense in which I use the term, refers neither to the actions of a calculating political subject, nor to the operations of bureaucratic mechanisms and personnel. It describes, rather, a certain way of striving to reach social and political ends by acting in a calculated manner upon the forces, activities and relations of the individuals that constitute a population.
>
> (Rose, 1989:4)

The framework I want to propose for understanding public health is that which sees it as one of the governmental techniques under which externally imposed authority and domination has progressively been replaced by techniques for governing internal life. The connection between, on the one hand, systems of power and domination, and on the other hand 'technologies of the self' whereby individuals seek to improve their capacities and conduct has been dubbed *governmentality* (Foucault, 1988:18). The concept of governmentality has attracted considerable attention in recent years (Foucault, 1979; Burchell, Gordon and Miller, 1991; Miller and Rose, 1990; Rose, 1989). Foucault proposed the term governmentality to describe the connection between on the one hand 'technologies of power, which determine the conduct of individuals and submit them to certain ends or domination, an objectivising of the subject' and on the other,

> technologies of the self, which permit individuals to effect by their own means or with the help of others a certain number of operations on their own bodies and souls, thoughts, conduct and way of being, so as to transform themselves in order to attain a certain state of happiness, purity, wisdom, perfection or immortality.
>
> (Foucault, 1988:18)

The Foucauldian concept of governmentality takes population as the target of power, and emphasizes the tactical deployment of governmental calculation.

There are two fundamental aspects to the operation of contemporary government. First, the target of power is populations. Second, power has tended to shift from the exercise of domination from outside, to the adoption of governmental aims by the subjects of power themselves. This latter tendency has characteristically worked through the mediation of expertise. New realms of life are continually being opened up to the exercise of expertise, principally of the various 'psy-disciplines', and so made amenable to governmental calculation.

The modern history of public health is consistent with, and a good illustration of, the governmentality thesis. The great public health developments of the nineteenth century were those which, using the new sciences of social statistics, categorized and inventorized the populations of the poor and marshalled sanitation and urban planning to the task of improving their conditions. In this century, the concerns with external health conditions are augmented by the development of a range of expertises in psychological health. Psychology becomes the vast new field of the twentieth century, applied to everything from industrial production to marriage guidance (Rose, 1989).

Governmentality and HIV/AIDS

HIV/AIDS can be situated within this general picture of the development of public health. Once it was recognized as a public health threat, HIV/AIDS, like any other new public health issue, became an issue of concern to government. For a number of reasons though HIV/AIDS has been a particularly intense site of governmental concerns. AIDS was not a biological irruption into an unstructured, natural field. HIV/AIDS has a history and a pre-history which has done more than determine the reception of a new biological entity — it has structured the way in which HIV/AIDS itself has been constituted.

Gay men created the conditions of possibility for AIDS. Were it not for the existence of this group as a discrete population, in which the unusual frequency of certain diseases could be noticed, then AIDS would not have been identified when it was. The circumstances of the construction of AIDS have had a number of consequences. One is the prominence of epidemiology in the definition and control of HIV/AIDS (Oppenheimer, 1992). Another is the centrality of the connection between homosexuality and AIDS. This connection accounts for the classification of AIDS as a sexually transmitted disease. It would be more appropriate to see HIV as a blood borne virus in the same way hepatitis is. But AIDS cannot shake off the circumstances of its discovery: appearing in a population constituted by its sexuality, it must be a sexually transmitted disease.

The government of HIV/AIDS has therefore involved the intersection of two intertwined governmental realms — those of public health and sexuality. This has had some perverse effects — the potential remedicalization of homosexuality for example, just when it seemed the battle against this had been won. But its main effect has been to strengthen those aspects of public health which concern the self-governing person. Prevailing contemporary norms are liberal in their attitude to consensual sexual expression, but in reality this freedom is undergirded by a network of laws and training which govern sexual conduct. The advent of HIV has led to an additional element in this range of issues in relation to sexual conduct, the need to protect against the risk of HIV infection. But prevailing methods of the government of sexual conduct do not lend themselves to externally imposed, top-down public health solutions, such as apply, for example, to vaccination programmes. The paradigmatic forms of public health in relation to sexual conduct are those which involve self-control and self-management. They are a subset of those public health concerns which have based themselves on the statistical identification of patterns of health outcomes among different sectors of the population and which have sought to devise risk reduction strategies for those populations at highest risk. The government of HIV/AIDS thus places the line between good and bad in a specific way.

> This assimilation of all behaviours that might increase risk and their opposition to risk avoiding behaviours changes the dividing line between the normal and the abnormal. The opposition is no longer the 'normal' majority heterosexual behaviour as opposed to perversity. The new dividing line separates the 'reasonable' (highly valued) from the 'irrational' (to be combated) in terms of the criterion of fatal risk. This is the basis for a redefinition of a hygienic approach to sexuality centred around conceptions of self-control and risk management.
>
> (Pollak, 1992:88)

The identification of a 'new' population at risk

Having sketched the framework for the notion of government in relation to HIV/AIDS, I want to turn to a specific example of government in this field, namely the creation of a particular type of person. To see this process at its most active, I will take the example of a population whose creation is very new. Over the past few years, a new object has been created as part of the international fight against the AIDS pandemic: the population of men who have sex with men. This population has variously been seen as a progressive vantage point from which to seek to ensure that resource allocation mirrors the real epidemiology of HIV and as a reactionary attempt on the part of health authorities to de-gay AIDS. I want to look at some of the logic according to which the population of men who have sex with men has been posited. On that basis I will suggest some of the ways in which it may be appropriate to react to this new population.

There are some accounts of HIV/AIDS policies which take as their starting point an essential opposition between homosexuality and the State. From this perspective, the association between HIV/AIDS and homosexuality, at least in the industrialized world, has determined national responses to the epidemic, resulting in an oscillation between indifference and repression. Advances in ameliorating the effects of the HIV/AIDS epidemic are credited to the heroic triumph of the gay community against entrenched State-homophobia. There is some truth to these accounts, and more so in some countries than others. In

Australia, the period of government indifference to AIDS was relatively short-lived, with less than two years between the first gay community discussions of this emerging new health threat and the first commitment to a nationally funded and co-ordinated AIDS strategy. From this time on, the Australian Government has recognized the role of gay men and of the gay community in facing the epidemic.

In other countries, the early AIDS policy history is not so positive. In both Britain and the US, right wing governments with moralistic agendas were unsympathetic to the public inclusion of gay men and gay community agendas in national AIDS policy making. Recent research has concluded that the distaste for gay sex and lack of sympathy to gay men of senior British Cabinet Ministers, including the then Prime Minister Thatcher, hampered AIDS education in Britain in the latter half of the 1980s (The Pink Paper, 1993; Miller and Williams, 1993). Notwithstanding significant national differences in the political reception of gay men and the gay community, the account of HIV/AIDS in terms of an essential opposition between homosexuality and the state is mistaken. This is especially so as HIV/AIDS has shifted from being a matter of political crisis, to be dealt with by short term measures decided at ministerial level, to a public health matter, the responsibility of the public health apparatus at all its governmental levels. I want now to turn to the question to exactly how HIV/AIDS ought to be situated in the context of public health.

In an interesting recent article, David Armstrong uses Mary Douglas' notion of the line between the polluted and the clean to discuss public health. He divides public health over the past two hundred years into four main periods:

Quarantine, which drew a line between places;

Sanitary science which guarded a line between the body and its natural environment;

Interpersonal hygiene which persuaded those same bodies to maintain a line between each other;

The new public health which deploys its lines of hygienic surveillance everywhere throughout the body politic.

(Armstrong, 1993:24)

From the period of interpersonal hygiene, issues of psychological health and individual difference start to become predominant. Techniques of public health shift from ways of persuading populations to protect themselves from ill health to providing populations with the means of reaching their full potential. This tendency is taken to new heights of sophistication with the new public health, which conceives of an interdependent relationship between individuals, communities and their social and political environment. Community development thus becomes the key strategy of the new public health.

Community development as a governmental health promotion technique requires that particular populations be identified as communities and that they be assisted to enhance their capacity to meet their goals, which amounts to their taking on governmental objectives for themselves. This process is mediated by expertise, in two ways. Particular experts in community development are created, for example, a gay community peer educator or an outreach worker, or the generic community development experts familiar to the overseas aid field. But as well, the new public health operates by assigning the notion of expertise to the community itself as a whole. That is, the idea that the community are the experts and must be consulted is not merely a piece of sloganeering on the part of disgruntled masses in the face of an unfeeling bureaucracy. It should be taken seriously as one of the key elements of the operation of public health.

The analysis of public health I am proposing suggests that the gay community finds its involvement in HIV/AIDS policy making not as a matter of defiance of the normal logic of government and public health, but as the consequence of this logic. It represents the triumph of good government rather than the triumph against government. In the space of the definition of populations, the specification of communities and the designation of particular expertises are continual contestations. Governments, bureaucracies, local administrations and community organizations all tug this way and that in the pursuit of their interests over these matters. One particular (perhaps key) point of contestation has arisen in the use of the term, and perhaps the creation of the population, of men who have sex with men.

Men who have sex with men

The domain of government with its attendant techniques of population, community and expertise is a limited domain. It does not and cannot encompass the full range of human behaviour, let alone come to grips with the operations of desire and the psyche. Given this limitation, there is always scope for the tactical extension of government into some hitherto ungoverned realm. The expression of male homosexual desire and male homosexual behaviour is not coextensive with gay identity or membership of the gay male community. In countries where a major route of transmission of HIV is sex between men, a legitimate public health question is: how adequate is the gay community as a means of reaching all men who have sex with men?

This sort of question has recently been posed by the Australian Government in research commissioned by the Department of Health in relation to approaches to HIV/AIDS education for men who have sex with men who do not identify as gay or with the gay community. This research project was recently completed by John McLeod, Phil Nott and me on behalf of the Australian Federation of AIDS Organizations, and I will now turn to discuss the results of this research in greater detail. I will use the acronym MSM, standing for 'men who have sex with men', to refer to men who have sex with men who do not identify as gay or who do not identify with the gay community. I use this acronym to distinguish this particular delimited category from those usages which refer to all men who have sex with men, including gay men.

There has been some controversy attached to the use of the term 'men who have sex with men', especially where the term is used in whole or in part to refer to gay men (Duffin, 1992; Pollak, 1992). Superficially, the dispute is about whether it is acceptable to use 'men who have sex with men' as a depoliticized euphemism for gay men. More substantially, however, the dispute concerns whether programmes will be conducted by public health authorities in the name of the population of men who have sex with men, or with and through the gay community (Bartos, 1993). I do not aim here to resolve this dispute. My use of MSM should not be taken to imply that the term 'men who have sex with men' can or should substitute for 'gay men' or 'gay community' where those terms are more relevant. However, it does imply that the identity gay man, or the community of gay men, does not encompass all men who have sex with men.

The genesis of the Australian Government's decision to commission a study of MSM came from two sources. First Australia's *National HIV/AIDS Strategy*, adopted in August 1989, argued that an effective HIV/AIDS education strategy must address both men who have sex with men who identify with the gay community and those who for reasons of identity (e.g. bisexual men), access or choice, do not identify with the gay community. This second group of men has been addressed in a number of ways. An outdoor and convenience advertising campaign which used short texts placed as advertisements on public transport, etc., included one story about a man who had sex with men and women; community-based organizations (and, more recently, two health authorities) have developed outreach programmes, particularly for men who use public places for sex with other men. However, the total effort directed at this group of men has been small.

Second, in 1990, in response to concerns about the continuing incidence of unsafe sex among homosexually active men, the Department of Health took up a proposal from Australia's largest community based non-government AIDS organization, the AIDS Council of New South Wales, to develop a national media campaign to encourage the continuation of safe sex practices. It was decided that this campaign should be in two parts, the first focusing on gay men and the second on MSM. A print and radio advertising campaign targeted at gay men ran between February and July 1991. While this campaign nominally targeted gay and bisexual men, in reality it was directed only at gay men.

Before undertaking a second stage campaign focusing on MSM, it was decided that a research study was needed to provide a qualitative picture and detailed insights into men in the target audience. Interviews were conducted with 97 men who have sex with men who do not identify as gay or with the gay community. Thirty-nine of these were lengthy face to face interviews. Men for these interviews were recruited by snowballing recruitment techniques, through contacts from mainly community sector service providers with a history of working with the target group. An additional 58 telephone interviews were conducted, in response to newspaper advertisements in Melbourne.

The men were not asked their HIV status, and none volunteered that they HIV positive. The majority lived in metropolitan areas, but significant numbers lived in regional centres or rural areas. Interviewees came from the Northern Territory, South Australia, Victoria, Tasmania, the ACT and Queensland. New South Wales, which is Australia's most populous state and the one with a large concentration of gay men, was not included on the grounds that extensive work with MSM had already taken place or was in progress in that State, and especially in the west of Sydney (Bennett, Chapman and Bray, 1989; O'Reilly, 1991; Davis, Klemmer and Dowsett, 1991; Sorrell, Crawford and O'Reilly, 1992). The substantive interviews were supplemented with interviews with service providers working with the target group, which also helped to put the findings in their policy context.

The long interviews with men from the target group concentrated on eliciting detailed information about episodes of unsafe sex, or sexual encounters where the decision to have safe or unsafe sex was difficult. It was decided to focus closely on episodes of unsafe sex because this has been an area inadequately dealt with in the past. Unsafe sex has become a fraught issue, especially for gay men. In part, this is a consequence of the successful formation of a safe sex culture. In many gay communities, safe sex norms have become widely disseminated and almost universally known. As many survey results can attest, the level of safe sex knowledge is almost universal among gay men, and the level of reported safe sex behaviour is also very high, especially in areas where the gay community is concentrated (Crawford *et al.*, 1992; Coates, 1990). This has had the perverse effect of making disclosure of episodes of unsafe sex difficult, especially for gay men (Odets, 1990).

Unfortunately, the discussion of unsafe sex has not been helped by the discourse of *relapse*. As a number of commentators have suggested, the relapse model is an inappropriate way of describing the failure to sustain safe sex because amongst other things it pathologizes unsafe sex (Bochow, 1992; Davies and Weatherburn, 1991). From this debate there has emerged a more sophisticated account of why it is gay men continue to have unsafe sex. Hart *et al.* (1992) propose that the investigation of unsafe sex needs to operate from the assumption that 'men have either made a decision to engage in a particular type of sexual behaviour, and thus accepted the risks involved, or have explicitly consented to its taking place.' In relation to gay men, this debate is being furthered by the examination of the issue of 'negotiated safety'. Our research study started from the premise that MSM continue to have unprotected anal intercourse because it feels good and is life affirming. In this respect, we expected MSM to be no different from gay men (Prieur, 1990; Pollak, 1992; Bochow, 1992). Given this starting point, the interviews were conducted in a way designed to elicit discussion of unsafe sex, by acknowledging the difficulties in always sustaining safe sex. We sought to dig beneath the pat recitation of safe sex rules which often characterizes responses to safe sex surveys.

I now turn to an examination of what it is possible to generalize about the nature of MSM. Then I look at the factors associated with their practice of unsafe sex, and how unsafe sex is experienced. I then consider the implications for HIV/AIDS education directed towards MSM. First, what can be generalized about MSM, notwithstanding that we know they are not a group of men of a particular type (Dowsett, 1991). Sexual identity is not a major issue for MSM. Sexuality is not a key part of their sense of personal identity, which is based instead on other personal relationships, such as family, career, etc. Some men in our study actively refused a gay sexual identity, for others it was simply irrelevant. Nor did these men think of themselves as bisexual, although if they had to choose a sexual identity, some were prepared to be called bisexual. Typical was the comment made to the interviewer: 'I suppose *you'd* call me bisexual'. The category of bisexual seems to be more an artefact of researchers of sexual behaviour than it is a real lived identity.

MSM also distinguish themselves from gay men. We found they did so on the basis of idiosyncratic and relatively arbitrary markers, for instance by not kissing the men they have sex with. The fact that these men see gay men as different from themselves has implications for the types of services they are prepared to access. For example, they tend to regard community based AIDS bodies as gay organizations and are therefore reluctant to approach them.

Our study found MSM to have very high levels of safe sex knowledge, which is consistent with the findings of the most recent large scale telephone survey of gay-attached and non-gay attached men who have sex with men in Australia, Project Male-Call (Crawford, *et al.*, 1992). But beyond basic safe sex knowledge, these MSM made fine gradations in their assessment of the risk of various sexual practices. Insertive anal intercourse and withdrawal before ejaculation were regarded as unsafe, but as less risky than unprotected receptive anal intercourse. This leads on to a second set of issues, which is what factors are associated with the practice of unsafe sex by MSM?

A majority of the MSM in our study had some history or current practice of unsafe sex (we defined unsafe sex as unprotected anal or vaginal intercourse). Unsafe sex was associated with isolation, assumptions about sexual partners, self esteem, the extent of anal orientation, comfort with condoms, and fatalism. A key issue for many MSM is that they are socially or geographically isolated from other men who have sex with men and from the HIV epidemic. HIV is not a reality in many of these men's lives. Their social isolation from the gay community is a powerful metaphor for their personal, physical isolation from the virus. The locational effects which have been observed in relation to gay men (Kippax *et al.*, 1990) are exacerbated by these men who do not identify as gay. These men made decisions to engage in unsafe sex on the basis of superficial characteristics of their sexual partners. They assumed that a partner outwardly similar to themselves, especially in standards of personal hygiene, would have the same HIV status. We also found that a number of MSM would have unsafe sex because their sexual partner did not seem to be gay. Somewhat different dynamics applied to unsafe sex between men of different cultural backgrounds or of very different ages. Here, unsafe sex was related to the assumption of stereotypically dominant and subordinate roles.

In general, risk assessments are being made by MSM in their decisions to have unsafe sex. Sexual partners will be chosen, sometimes with great discrimination at other times with less discrimination. Some of these strategies are plausible — negotiated safety with one partner of known HIV status — but others are clearly foolhardy — avoidance of dirty partners. The quality of that decision-making process is mediated by a variety of factors.We found that for a significant number of MSM, a fatalistic attitude operates as a mediator of their risk assessments. Fatalism inclined some men to adopt optimistic assessments of the risk of unsafe sex.

High self esteem was also positively related to the decision to have safe sex, and the converse for low self esteem and unsafe sex. Self esteem tended to be a particular problem for the younger men and those from non-Anglo backgrounds in our study. Some self-esteem building strategies in relation to HIV have relied on making men feel good about their gay identities. These would be entirely misplaced in this target group. Strategies for increasing self esteem should not assume that MSM must be put on a track to coming out as gay. Identity and self-esteem issues come together in the case of MSM who also have sex with women. This group has been the subject of attention as presenting a major HIV risk to women (and the subject of inappropriate attention as a potential 'threat to the whole community', as if transmission among exclusively homosexual men is tolerable). We found there was a strong tendency for MSM who are protective of relationships with wives and children to have exclusively safe sex with other men. Because the fear of 'bringing something home' is a powerful motivator to have exclusively safe sex with other men, the relationship with a female partner should be regarded as a positive attribute for those men who have sex with both men and women. It therefore follows that educational strategies which might have the unintended consequence of disrupting the relationship between these men and their female partners, such as encouraging MSM to give up sex with women, or educating women to recognize signs that their male partner may also be having sex with men, should not be supported.

As well as these characteristics of the affective context in which MSM have unsafe sex, there are some more immediately physical variables in the likelihood of unsafe sex taking place. Not all MSM are anally-oriented in their sexual preferences. Unsafe sex is always going to be an important and difficult issue for those men who tend to prefer anal sex. Men whose anal orientation is less important are much more willing and find it easier to adopt safe sex. Pleasure in anal intercourse depends on a successful initiation into anal eroticism. We found that rimming (oral-anal sex) is a powerful way of establishing anal eroticism, and rimming will often be followed by anal intercourse.

Another more physical factor related to condom use. Many men reported they are reluctant to use condoms because they find them uncomfortable, or that they make it hard to sustain an erection. More important, though, is that condoms are perceived as an interruption to the natural flow of sex, which leads to a third set of issues, namely how do MSM experience unsafe sex?

The ethnographic methodology of the study lent itself to a discussion of the symbolic significance of unsafe sex. Detailed notes of what the men had to say, in their words, formed the basis for this analysis. It clearly emerged that many MSM have anal intercourse as a way of signifying the encounter or relationship is special. In order to heighten the intimacy of this contact, the sex is often unsafe. Unsafe sex functions as the consummation of a relationship. It is associated with feelings of love and security. Anal intercourse is experienced as time out of time, because of its singularity, its intensity and because it represents the Other of everyday life.

These MSM often experience their sex with other men outside the context of their other social relationships. It is constructed as a particular relationship with another, special man. They will be impervious to safe sex education which places sexual behaviour in the context of a sexual community, because they do not see themselves as part of such a community. MSM do not see themselves as belonging to a particular group. This creates challenges for the way in which the targeting of educational strategies is conceptualized. Targeting can be reductionist, focusing on smaller and smaller groups of people. The tendency is for targeting to be conceived of as the precise specification of a discrete audience to which the educational message should be delivered. We prefer the notion of an audience's engagement with the message, as an active and interactive process. It is preferable to reconceptualize targeting as engagement, where education strategies seek to engage with people on the basis of what they have in common.

Health education for MSM

HIV/AIDS education which relies purely on an audience accepting the simple message of safe sex every time does not encourage the audience to bring something of their own experience of the ambiguity of safe sex decision making to interact with the health promotion message. This didacticism belies the quite complex personal risk assessment and risk reduction strategies which are presently being used by men to avoid HIV infection.

The key issue we found in MSM's experience of unsafe sex was that they had no social context for this sex — it was a matter of a particular occasion, with a special man. Given this, the task of HIV/AIDS education for these men needs to be to find ways of allowing these men to place their sex with other men in a wider context. HIV/AIDS health promotion needs to normalize sex between men. As well, given their isolation from the epidemic, HIV and its consequences needs to be brought home, in a straightforward and sensitive manner without being designed to shock or horrify. Health promotion approaches should build on the already high levels of knowledge in the community about the basic facts of HIV transmission. They should embed the safe sex message in the context of sexual negotiation, relationships, places and circumstances. They need to address the logic of the risk assessment strategies which MSM use to make decisions about safe or unsafe sex. Where the reasoning in these risk assessment strategies is flawed, these flaws should be exposed.

A major way in which the context of sexual activity can be emphasized is through the use of personal narratives. Radio is an appropriate medium for the delivery of these narratives because its format is suited to relatively extended narrative, it is cheap and accessible for listeners, and because the messages can be listened to unobtrusively. Unlike some of the strategies which appear to have been successful within the gay community, eroticizing the safe sex message is not a useful strategy for MSM. Given these considerations, what is the best framework for the development and delivery of HIV/AIDS education for MSM?

Since 1984, HIV/AIDS education in Australia has been pursued in a community health framework. The early experience, especially of Health Minister Neal Blewett, of the successes of the San Francisco Model (Coates, 1990) was translated into national policy and has guided Australia's national strategy on HIV/AIDS since. The community focus, and the explicit partnership between communities, the medical profession and governments is widely credited as a major factor in Australia's relative success in minimizing the spread and ameliorating the effects of HIV (National Evaluation, 1992). However, translating this community emphasis into programmes directed towards MSM will not be easy.

Given that there are few community-based agencies which deal with sexuality, inevitably the main bodies which will be willing to address issues around sex between men are the community AIDS bodies which are used to dealing with gay men's issues. However, there needs to be a greater effort to bring MSM within the focus of community based gay oriented AIDS organizations. Existing outreach programmes should be extended, but the presentation of the services of AIDS organizations and their publicly promoted education materials should also include MSM. Given that many MSM want to talk about their experiences, telephone counselling services appropriate to their needs are an important strategy.

While community-based organizations are likely to remain the focus of concentrated programmes for MSM, other agencies should also be encouraged to take up these issues. Health care settings are an important way in which issues of sexual health can be raised for MSM. Services need to become more skilled at being open to the possibility that men who are not gay may nevertheless have sex with other men. A long term strategy should be to place HIV within the context of men's health and men's sexual health.

It is possible to develop educational strategies which engage men who have sex with men who do not identify as gay or with the gay community. This engagement needs to work with these men, and neither try to turn them into gay men nor discourage them from having sex with other men. The only possibility of grappling with HIV for these men is if their sexual activity can be acknowledged as a discrete *and* discreet part of their lives. Our study found that MSM are able to separate their sexual activity from the rest of their sense of personal identity, and this separation was an aid to their adoption of safe sex. The fact that most of these men clearly separate their sexual activity from the rest of their lives suggests that it would be mistaken to work through community agencies such as youth groups, ethnic community organizations, sporting clubs, etc., to reach these men. What is needed are greater opportunities for direct outreach to these men, access to telephone information and counselling services appropriate to their needs, widely disseminated but low key media strategies which normalize sex between men, and a greater preparedness on the part of health care providers to admit the possibility that all sorts of men may have sex with other men.

While we stand by the conclusion of our study that it would be counter-productive to deliver HIV/AIDS education to MSM through ethnic minority community organizations which do not currently deal with homosexuality, there is one qualification which needs to be added. The meanings of sex between men *within* particular ethnic or cultural minority groups may be quite different from the meanings *across* cultures. For that subject to be fully explored, we will need studies designed to operate within particular groups, and conducted by members of that same group. The minority of men from non-Anglo backgrounds who were interviewed for this project indicated that they view sex with other men from their own background differently from the way they regard sex with Anglo men. Not surprisingly, they were not prepared to go into those differences in the context of this project. Nevertheless, even for these men, there was common ground with Anglo men in the way in which they saw their own sexual activity.

We need to ensure that the voices of MSM are better heard. Over the past few years, the value of gay community attachment has become a touchstone of Australian HIV/AIDS education efforts, but the story does not end there. There are men who have sex with men who are perfectly happy in their sexual activity, but who do not see themselves as gay and have no interest in the gay community. These men need a clearer voice so that programmes which meet their needs can be devised and delivered within a community framework. This work also needs to come to terms with the good reasons men are continuing to have unsafe sex. In this regard, it may be useful to bear in mind that men who have sex with men who do not identify as gay continue to have unsafe sex for reasons which may apply just as powerfully to gay men.

Conclusion

The arguments advanced in this Australian study of MSM who do not identify as gay or with the gay community suggest it is a population which can be worked with, and not necessarily to the detriment of continuing work with gay men. But the question I have not yet answered is: what is driving the creation of the population of men who have sex with men and is it a force which should be resisted? There are at least three vantage points from which the creation of the population of men who have sex with men can be seen.

One is as a strategy to 'de-gay' HIV/AIDS, by replacing a community defined category with one defined by health and population professionals. The second is to invoke the population as a site of danger, where good, educable gay men are contrasted with men who have sex with men as pure vectors of transmission from the homosexual to the heterosexual population. The third vantage point sees men who have sex with men as a conceptual and administrative category to enable the extension of the government of sex between men.

I suggested above that although community development is an orthodox public health strategy, it is always subject to contestation. Public health strategies abound with examples of bureaucratically defined populations to which health programmes are, largely unsuccessfully, delivered. The management of community development programmes is a complex and sometimes unpredictable task from a core bureaucracy point of view. Administrative requirements may be more easily met by defining and attempting to measure a population of men who have sex with men, rather than managing the politics of gay community development. In contrast to an administratively defined, and contained, population, the population of men who have sex with men can also be invoked as a space of unconstrained danger. Returning to the points made by David Armstrong above, one aspect of Mary Douglas' work he develops is the notion of the dividing line between the pure and the polluted, a line which in effect defines the social by containing it. Armstrong suggests that as public health has progressed, this line has become a space of greater volume, and risk and danger lie within that line/space. In other words, the space between healthy and unhealthy is a space of ungovernment. Men who have sex with men represent the dangerous, ungoverned and ungovernable exercise of desire, which threatens to pollute society. It is notable that the media demonization of 'bisexual men putting their innocent wives at risk of AIDS' seems to have a greater currency than plain old-fashioned homophobic demonization. Similarly, the public policy interest in men who have sex with men has often been expressed as a concern for the female partners of bisexual men, in a way which implies that the men themselves and their male partners are expendable. Both the argument for paying attention to men who have sex with men on grounds of the supremacy of administrative bureaucracy and on grounds of avoiding the danger of pollution should, in my view, be opposed.

However, there does remain one point of view from which men who have sex with men should be the subject of attention, and that is the extension of the scope of government of sex between men. For this to be able to happen in the ways I have suggested above, there will need to be a dissociation between notions of community and those of identity. In other words, ways will need to be found of publicly affirming the positive experience of sex between men, on the assumption that any man is able to have such an experience. It would place men who have sex with men within the bounds of community. If this proves possible, it will represent a significant reshaping of the contours of that space between the social and the ungoverned, the pure and the polluted.

References

ARMSTRONG, D. (1993) 'Public health spaces and the fabrication of identity', *Sociology*, 27, 3.

BARTOS, M. (1993) 'Governing AIDS', *Australian Left Review*, 148, March.

BENNETT, G. CHAPMAN, S. and BRAY, F. (1989) 'Sexual practices and beats: AIDS-related sexual practices in a sample of homosexual and bisexual men in the western area of Sydney', *Medical Journal of Australia*, 151.

BOCHOW, M. (1992) 'Determinants of risk-taking behaviour', paper presented at the 8th International Conference on AIDS, Amsterdam.

BURCHELL, G., GORDON, C. and MILLER, P. (1991) (Eds) *The Foucault Effect studies in governmentality*, London: Harvester Wheatsheaf.

COATES, T.J. (1990) 'Strategies for modifying sexual behaviour for primary and secondary prevention of HIV disease', *Journal of Consulting and Clinical Psychology*, 58, 1.

CRAWFORD, J., KIPPAX, S., RODDEN, P. and BENTON, K. (1992) *Preliminary Report on Project Male-Call, National Telephone Survey of Men who have Sex with Men*, Sydney, National Centre for HIV Social Research (Macquarie University Unit).

DAVIES, P. and WEATHERBURN, P. (1991) 'Towards a general model of sexual negotiation', in AGGLETON, P., HART, G. and DAVIES, P. (Eds) *AIDS: Responses, Interventions and Care*, London: The Falmer Press.

DAVIS, M., KLEMMER, U. and DOWSETT, G. (1991) *Bisexually Active Men and Beats: Theoretical and Educational Implications*, Sydney: AIDS Council of NSW and Macquarie University AIDS Research Unit.

DOWSETT, G. (1991) *Men who have Sex with Men: Considerations for a National HIV/AIDS Educational Intervention*, Canberra: Commonwealth Department of Health, Housing and Community Services.

DUFFIN, R. (1992) 'People with HIV and the National Conference', *National AIDS Bulletin*, December/January 1993.

FOUCAULT, M. (1979) 'Governmentality', *Ideology & Consciousness*, 6.

FOUCAULT, M. (1988) 'Technologies of the self', in MARTIN, L.H., GUTMAN, H. and HUTTON, P.H. (Eds) *Technologies of the Self, A Seminar with Michel Foucault*, London: Tavistock

HART, G., BOULTON, M., FITZPATRICK, R., MCLEAN, J. and DAWSON, J. (1992) '"Relapse" to unsafe sexual behaviour among gay men: A critique of recent behavioural HIV/AIDS research', *Sociology of Health and Illness*, 14, 2.

KIPPAX, S., CRAWFORD, J., CONNELL, R.W., DOWSETT, G.W., WATSON, L., RODDEN, P., BAXTER, D. and BERG, R. (1990) *The Importance of Gay Community in the Prevention of HIV Transmission*, Social Aspects of the Prevention of AIDS Study A — Report No 7, Sydney: Macquarie University.

MILLER, D. and WILLIAMS, K. (1993) 'From icebergs and tombstones to personal testimony: The AIDS public education campaign, 1986–90', Abstract at the Seventh Conference on Social Aspects of AIDS, London.

MILLER, P. and ROSE, N. (1990) 'Governing economic life', *Economy and Society*, 19, 1.

NATIONAL EVALUATION (1992) 'Report of the evaluation of the national HIV/AIDS strategy', report to the Minister for Health, Housing and Community Services and the Intergovernmental Committee on AIDS by the National Evaluation Steering Committee, Canberra.

O'REILLY, C. (1991) 'Western Sydney Men who have sex with men project', Western Sydney AIDS Unit, Western Sydney Area Health Service, Sydney.

ODETS, W. (1990) *The Psychological Impact: The Impact of AIDS on Uninfected Gay and Bisexual Men*, privately circulated.

OPPENHEIMER, G.M. (1992) 'Causes, cases and cohorts: The role of epidemiology in the historical construction of AIDS', in FEE, E. and FOX, D.M. (Eds) *AIDS: The Making of a Chronic Disease*, Berkeley, CA: University of California Press.

THE PINK PAPER (1993) 'Thatcher's Distate', **284**, 2 July, 28.

POLLAK, M. (1992) 'AIDS: A problem for sociological research', *Current Sociology*, **40**, 3.

PRIEUR, A. (1990) 'Norwegian gay men: Reasons for continued practice of unsafe sex', *AIDS Education and Prevention*, **2**, 2.

ROSE, N. (1989) *Governing the soul: The shaping of the private self*, London: Routledge.

SIMEY, T.S. (1937) *Principles of Social Administration*, London: Oxford University Press.

SORRELL, T.S., CRAWFORD, J. and O'REILLY, C.G. (1992) 'Non-gay identified homosexually active men targeting strategies identification project (project abstract)', *HIV/AIDS Research*, Department of Health, Housing and Community Services, Australian Government Publishing Service, Canberra, September.

Chapter 7

Assimilating Safer Sex: Young Heterosexual Men's Understanding of 'Safer Sex'

Daniel Wight

The term *safer sex* has been used since the mid-1980s in British HIV/AIDS health education, superseding the earlier phrase *safe sex* which health educators considered less accurate. Nearly all surveys of young people confirm that they have a high level of knowledge about the main transmission routes of HIV (McEwan and Bhopal, 1991, Wight, 1993a). However, their precise understanding of the term safer sex has received little attention, beyond establishing widespread knowledge of the prophylactic value of condoms. This seems to be an important omission given the frequency with which safer sex is advocated without any explication. One of the few surveys that have investigated this topic questioned 879 18-year-olds in the Glasgow area (Macintyre and West, 1993), using a question designed and subsequently used by the National Survey of Sexual Attitudes and Lifestyles (Johnson *et al.*, 1994). This chapter reinterprets these survey findings using qualitative data from detailed interviews with 58 19-year-old Glaswegian men. By analysing young men's responses in relation to the wider social context of their sexual beliefs and behaviour it can be seen how the term safer sex has been assimilated into their pre-existing construction of sexuality.

National health education campaigns and mass media coverage of HIV/AIDS have been vague about what constitutes safer sex. The leaflet *Don't Die of Ignorance*, delivered to every household in Britain in 1987, used the phrase once, in a heading: 'Use condoms for safer sex'. There was no mention of non-penetrative sex other than the (bracketed) information that: 'It could also be that oral sex can be risky particularly if semen is taken into the mouth.' In this early stage of the campaign, television advertisements exhorted the public to 'protect' themselves, and the only reference to safer sex was: 'It's safer if you use a condom.' The campaign was clearly predicated on the norm of penetrative vaginal intercourse, thus reproducing dominant heterosexuality (Wilton and Aggleton, 1991). In contrast, most of the safer sex advertising for gay men at that time discouraged penetration (Hart, 1993).

Subsequently the campaign for heterosexuals was slightly modified as a result of feminist criticism within the Health Education Authority (Miller and Williams, forthcoming). A press campaign from December 1988 to March 1989 gave more detail about safer sex in the small print beneath the main picture, though it was less than explicit. For instance, 'But safer sex doesn't just mean fewer sexual partners. It also means using a condom, or even (sic) having sex that avoids penetration.' In the 1990 television campaign in which medical experts encouraged people to 'protect yourselves' there was no mention of safer sex.

A study of British and Scottish national newspapers found that between 1988 and 1990 there were many references to *safe* or *safer sex* but very few to the specific behaviours which constitute safer sex (Bloor *et al.*, 1991). Out of nearly two thousand items on HIV/AIDS only 2 mentioned non-penetrative sex or masturbation and 3 oral sex, while the generic term 'body fluids' was often used in preference to explicit words like semen and vaginal secretions.

On network television the three most common AIDS stories covered on the news from 1986 to 1990 were the official government AIDS campaign, people living with HIV or AIDS, and reports on AIDS in other countries (Miller and Beharrell, 1993). Although the news coverage repeatedly criticized the educational campaign for its lack of explicit terminology, it never attempted to correct this omission (Miller and Williams, 1993). Detailed television coverage of the HIV-related risks of specific sexual activities was almost entirely restricted to documentaries and Thames Television's annual AIDS information series of 5 or 6 short episodes shown in the late evening (AIDS Help, AIDS Now, AIDS Update, etc.).

Probably the first survey data on what young people understand by safe sex were collected through two open-ended questions in 1987 with 200 14- and 15-year-old London school children (White *et al.*, 1988). Given the vagueness of publicly available messages on how to reduce the risk of transmitting HIV sexually, it was perhaps unsurprising that reported understanding of the phrase safe sex was limited primarily to condom use (83 per cent) and few partners (63 per cent). Oral and anal sex were mentioned in roughly similarly low numbers, both being considered *un*safe (6 per cent and 8 per cent respectively).

In 1990 a wide-ranging longitudinal survey of health and lifestyles, the West of Scotland Twenty-07 Study, asked 879 18-year-olds in the Glasgow area: 'There has been a lot of publicity about AIDS in the last year. What does the phrase "safer sex" mean to you?' The question was left open-ended in order to elicit respondent's own understandings, and interviewers prompted 'Anything else?' until the respondent said 'No'. Possible answers were listed on the schedule for the interviewers to tick.

The Glaswegian 18-year-olds appeared to have much the same understanding of safer sex that London 14- and 15-year olds had three years earlier. Eighty-five per cent of respondents mentioned condoms, 49 per cent fewer partners or only one, 36 per cent some aspect of partner choice, and only 2 per cent mentioned abstaining from specific sexual activities (Macintyre and West, 1993). Seven per cent said they did not know what safer sex meant, and 2 per cent referred to contraception other than condoms. There were few gender differences other than women more frequently mentioning monogamy or abstinence, a pattern previously identified (Rocheron and Linne, 1989). Further details of these findings and their social correlates can be found elsewhere (Macintyre and West, 1993).

Between May 1990 and the end of 1991 the National Survey of Sexual Attitudes and Lifestyles asked the same question of 4665 16–59-year-olds throughout Britain. The findings were similar to those obtained in the Glasgow survey, both for 16–24-year-olds and for the whole age range (Johnson *et al.*, 1994). However, fewer respondents mentioned condoms (78 per cent of 16–24-year-olds), many more mentioned the use of other contraception (14 per cent of 16–24-year-olds) and more than twice as many referred to abstaining from specific sexual practices (5 per cent of 16–24-year-olds).

The qualitative data presented below suggest that young Glaswegian men have a fuller understanding of safer sex than that elicited in the Twenty-07 Study and the National Survey, and they demonstrate how different research methods produce different findings. More generally, they show how young heterosexual men made sense of a new health education message by interpreting it in the light of their pre-existing construction of sexuality.

Methods

Fifty-eight 19-year-old men were recruited by subsampling from the youth cohort of the West of Scotland Twenty-07 Study. All male participants were approached in three contiguous postcode sectors on the edge of Glasgow, an area of council housing broadly similar to the city's other peripheral estates. The population is predominantly manual working class and overwhelmingly white. The young men had previously been contacted three times as part of the Twenty-07 Study (two face-to-face questionnaires, one postal), and due largely to survey loyalty, a response rate of 85 per cent was achieved. One respondent stated that he is gay.

I (male, married and heterosexual) interviewed respondents in depth for two to three hours in the first half of 1991. Everyone agreed to be audio-tape recorded, and nearly all chose to be interviewed in their homes. The topics covered included family, residence and employment history, friendship groups and leisure activities, learning about sex, early relationships with girls and detailed accounts of sexual histories. In order to explore the salience of HIV, the research was presented to potential respondents as a study of young men's lifestyles, friendships and sexual behaviour, and questions specific to HIV/AIDS were only asked in the last stage of the interview.

Amongst the issues raised concerning HIV, respondents were asked whether they knew the phrase safer sex and what it meant to them. Most respondents were probed to elicit whether they thought it related to HIV/AIDS, all sexually transmitted diseases and/or contraception. They were also questioned about their understanding of the relative HIV risks of oral, vaginal and anal sex. Their understanding of strategies by which to have safer sex was not only deduced from responses to these questions, but also from the sexual histories they had previously recounted. For instance, several described a strategy of partner choice (avoiding 'slags' and 'junkies') in relating their sexual experiences but did not mention this as a possible meaning of safer sex.

Results

The vast majority of respondents said safer sex means using a condom. Some stated 'use a contraceptive' or 'protection', but it seems likely that by this they meant use condoms. For instance:

> *DW*:   So what is it keeping you safe from?
> *Michael*: Initially I would say AIDS. I would also say unwanted pregnancy.
>   They are really the only two things that contraception can protect
>   you from. . .
> *DW*:   So if I say how do you have safer sex what would you say?
> *Michael*: Use a condom.

or

> *DW*:   What does that [safer sex] mean to you?
> *Tony*:   Contraception — condoms.

or

> *Kevin*:   Safer sex. Aye, I've heard that phrase.
> *DW*:   What does that mean to you?
> *Kevin*:   Using protection.
> *DW*   . . . when you're talking about safer sex you mean safer in relation
>   to?
> *Kevin*:   Well, if it's safer against AIDS I would say it's condoms . . .

Of the six men who did not mention condoms in discussing safer sex, five clearly demonstrated their knowledge of the prophylactic value of condoms in other parts of the interview. Only one of the fifty-eight respondents showed no awareness that condoms prevent HIV transmission.

Over half the sample had a broader concept of the sexual risks that the term safer sex referred to than simply HIV. Equal numbers of respondents thought the phrase covered pregnancy and all sexually transmitted diseases (STDs), most of them considering it applied to both. For instance:

DW: So do you think it [safer sex] is about diseases in general?

Gary: Well not just diseases, like if you are having sex like with a girl stopping her from getting pregnant. It doesn't just mean diseases. Condoms were out before diseases.

In contrast to the survey question used in the Twenty-07 Study (Macintyre and West, 1993) and the National Survey (Johnson *et al.*, 1994), in the in-depth interviews half the sample showed some knowledge of the relative HIV risks of different sexual behaviours. Of this group, most knew there is less risk of transmission from oral sex than either vaginal or anal sex, and half knew that anal sex carries greater risk than vaginal sex. However, only one person volunteered this information when questioned about safer sex without it being specifically sought.

While several respondents reported knowing nothing about the relative risks of different sexual behaviours, a third of the sample held incorrect views (judged by contemporary medical opinion). Thus 7 thought all three forms of sex equally likely to transmit the virus, 5 thought vaginal sex the least risky and, most worrying, 7 thought anal sex less risky than vaginal sex.

Understanding of safer sex was analysed in relation to perceived vulnerability to HIV and the readiness with which the disease was associated with gay men, but in neither case was any pattern discernible. As regards behaviour, those who reported more lifetime sexual partners were rather more likely to be knowledgeable about the relative risks of different sexual practices and to have a broader concept of what safer sex refers to, beyond HIV. There was some association between the reported practice of oral sex and knowing the relative risks of different sexual behaviours. Those who reported they had never engaged in oral sex were unaware that it is of relatively minor consequence for HIV transmission. Two men reported having engaged in heterosexual anal intercourse; one knew the relative HIV risks of anal, vaginal and oral sex, the other has learning difficulties and was the only respondent with wildly unorthodox views about AIDS, namely that it does not exist and has been fabricated by the government.

The assimilation of safer sex into the pre-existing construction of sexuality

Respondents' understanding of safer sex was congruent with their broader cultural construction of sexuality. The fact that half the sample thought, however vaguely, that safer sex refers to contraception and/or other STDs as well as HIV, reflected lay perceptions of sexual risks. HIV had very little importance in most of these young men's lives (Wight, 1993b), in contrast to the threat of unwanted pregnancy which led three-fifths always to practise contraception (after their first sexual intercourse). Large scale surveys confirm the salience of pregnancy for young people in contrast to that of HIV infection (Health Education Authority/MORI, 1990, Ford, 1991). Although few respondents had experienced STDs (in nearly all cases pubic lice), more knew people who had been infected; this was generally considered more probable than infection from HIV, though far less serious. Given the current shift amongst practitioners from HIV-specific health education for heterosexuals to a broader approach to sexual health, it is important to note that some young people have always understood safer sex in this more generic sense without it having much effect on their behaviour.

The primary meaning of sex for respondents was penetrative vaginal intercourse. This was apparent throughout the interviews and particularly evident when respondents were asked about their 'first sexual experience of *any kind*' which almost always prompted a description of their first experience of sexual intercourse. Sometimes other sexual practices were clearly distinguished from sex:

> *George*: Then we did not have sex then, it was about another week or two before we did. . .
> *DW*: And that first night, was it just kissing?
> *George*: She masturbated me.
> *DW*: To orgasm?
> *George*: Yeah.

In discussing non-penetrative sex the conversations below were not untypical:

> *DW*: So apart from using a condom is there other ways of having safer sex?
> *Shuggie*: What do you mean by that?
> *DW*: Well like —
> *Shuggie*: Have sex but not actually have sex?
> *DW*: Aye
> *Shuggie*: Is that what you are talking about? Like, have sex but not, like, putting it inside the lassie? Aye, I know what you are talking about now, aye.

or

> *Michael*: . . . Like how can it be safer sex when it is not sex?
> *DW*: So what is your definition?

Michael: My definition of sex is sexual intercourse.
DW: Which is?
Michael: The penis entering the vagina.

Given this meaning of sex (found elsewhere in Britain amongst both heterosexual men and women: Spencer, Faulkner and Keegan, 1988; Holland *et al.*, 1991), it is predictable that people should think of safer sex in terms of safer ways to have penetrative vaginal intercourse. This probably explains, as Macintyre and West suggested (1993), why only 2 per cent of Twenty-07 Study and 5 per cent of the National Survey respondents mentioned examples of non-penetrative sex when describing what 'safer sex' meant to them. Although half the 19-year-old men interviewed had some understanding of the relative risk for HIV of different sexual behaviours, this was only demonstrated when they were specifically questioned on the topic, not when asked what safer sex meant to them.

For the young men the restricted interpretation of safer sex was further exacerbated by the enormous symbolic significance vaginal intercourse has in their world. To a large extent this stems from the predominantly male context in which the men's concepts of sexuality had developed throughout their teens (Wight, in press). The compulsion to lose their virginity was an important component of their masculine ideology (cf. Spencer, 1984), and there was a great deal of speculation about the veracity of boys' claims to have experienced vaginal intercourse. Anything short of vaginal intercourse was insufficient to attain non-virgin status, however much erotic experience was gained. Whether or not one had 'done it' was seen by many to reflect one's ability to exert one's will over a girl (Wight, in press). This masculine esteem was further increased by seducing subsequent partners into having vaginal intercourse. Again, one act of vaginal intercourse was the critical criterion of having 'had' one's partner, not other forms of sex, however adventurous, or the duration of one's sexual relationship. The symbolic importance of vaginal intercourse for these young men reflects its meaning in British culture more widely, certainly as expressed in law: vaginal intercourse is central to the definition of rape, and, in England, lack of 'consummation' is grounds for annulment of marriage.

The significance of vaginal intercourse did not arise entirely from the masculine perspective of the young men's heterosexuality. As Kent *et al.* (1990) found, within affectionate heterosexual relationships initial vaginal intercourse was often regarded, by young women as well as men, as the culmination of a process of increasing intimacy, 'the final step, the last boundary'. 'For many people, having sexual intercourse seemed to be the final disambiguating step: we really are having a relationship. For others, it is confirmation of that relationship.' (Kent *et al.*, 1990:4)

The limited extent to which the young men discussed HIV/AIDS further reinforced their restricted interpretation of safer sex. Very few reported discussing the disease at any length with their parents or siblings, and most said they only rarely mentioned it with friends. When pushed to give examples of such occasions they usually described a pal being ridiculed for exposing himself to infection. His behaviour would prompt comments reiterating the need to wear condoms or select one's partners carefully, which were perhaps expressions of anxiety about AIDS:

> *DW*: And would you ever talk to them about AIDS?
> *Anthony*: No. Something that just doesn't crop up.
> *DW*: Would you talk to them about using condoms?
> *Anthony*: Occasionally, yes.
> *DW*: What kind of context?
> *Anthony*: I mean basically he'd turn round and say, 'I met this thing last night and then I slept with her.' 'Did you wear anything?'. 'No.' 'How no?' He says, 'I know, I know!' sort of thing, and that's the way it would come up.

or

> *DW*: Do you talk about it at all with your mates?
> *Ian*: No.
> *DW*: Do you ever joke about it?
> *Ian*: Oh aye.
> *DW*: Can you think of any examples of the way you might joke about it?
> *Ian*: Just if somebody gets off with one of the slags and he has not used contraception or anything. You are all slagging him and that, like, 'You have got AIDS' and 'You had better go for a check up' and that.

Very few of the young men interviewed reported talking about their sexual behaviour in any detail with their friends, beyond saying whether or not they were having vaginal intercourse.

Given the heterosexual construction of sexuality, safer sex was effectively assimilated as the use of condoms in penetrative vaginal sex. However, to a large extent respondents' understanding of which behaviours constituted 'safer sex' was irrelevant, since their predominant strategy to avoid HIV infection was to avoid infected partners. Only one man reported a sexual relationship with someone whom he thought might be HIV-positive, which he restricted to fondling and fellatio. The vast majority of the sample would not consider a sexual encounter with anyone thought to be infected:

> *DW*: Can you think of any occasion when you have not gone with a girl, or you have done something differently because of thinking about AIDS?

Mark: I don't think so. If I have had a chance like that I would stop it right away. If I ever meet anybody and you get that chance I would never do it, because of the fact I would not feel secure with them. I would not even go out with the person or anything like that, you know. I would just stop it there and then.

The young men's strategy of partner choice has been analysed elsewhere (Wight, 1993b). In short, their perception of risk and avoidance of unprotected vaginal intercourse was largely shaped by their perceived proximity to risk groups, defined as drug injectors, gay men, 'cows' or 'slags', and 'people from Edinburgh'. Of the 53 out of 58 who reported having had vaginal intercourse, a simple classification can be made between those who: i) reported no behavioural change because they were not concerned about HIV; ii) had not been concerned about HIV with partners to date and/or avoided risky partners; iii) avoided risky partners but if unsure avoided unprotected sex (usually by using condoms); and iv) were concerned about HIV with all potential partners and tried to use condoms until they knew them.

However, HIV was rarely of immediate salience in the choice of partners. Drug injectors and 'cows' were seen as polluting irrespective of the possibility of HIV, both being described as dirty and classed at the bottom of the hierarchy of working class respectability. In the case of drug injectors, respondents would not consider sexual contact with them.

So far as the young men were concerned, non-penetrative sex was primarily intended as a prelude or an accompaniment to penetrative intercourse, not as an alternative. About two-thirds of the sample had practised oral sex occasionally and about a further quarter did so frequently. This was often within long term relationships and in both directions. A minority of respondents discussed non-penetrative sex as a long term option. They were generally negative about it, either because it was perceived as less satisfying for them, or for their partners, or because it was not simultaneously pleasurable for both partners. There was some suggestion, however, that if it involved orgasm it might be a satisfactory substitute for penetrative sex:

Shuggie: I could get into it. I think any other guy could an' all. If a bird was at least going to do that to him it is not as if he is, not getting left out . . . Well he is still getting it really. Like still, fucking, into his balls.

The young men's girlfriends, on the other hand, were said to commonly veto penetrative sex, their main reported rationales being fear of conceiving or a wish to protect their reputation. Parallel research with a female subsample of the Twenty-07 Study, of the same age in the same cultural milieu, found that expressing these concerns may also have been a strategy to keep to non-penetrative sex for their own pleasure (Kitzinger, 1993).

It is worth noting that the primary meaning of sex, the significance of penetrative intercourse and the main context in which HIV was mentioned with friends was consistent across the sample. This is despite considerable variations in the young men's reported sexual histories, perceived vulnerability to HIV and the discourses they used to discuss sexuality. The central role of penetrative intercourse was so fundamental to these men's sexuality that it was common across their various sub-cultures.

Conclusion: social transformation or social control?

Of late there has been increasing discussion about the extent to which health promotion constitutes a new form of social regulation (e.g. Davies, 1991; Bunton, 1992). The involvement of health promotion in more and more areas of our everyday lives, whether or not we consider ourselves healthy, legitimates increasing surveillance of behaviours previously regarded as private — this publicly funded research on young men's sexual behaviour being a good case in point. Even an 'empowerment model' of health promotion can be regarded, in a Foucauldian sense, as a subtle technique of control, since it 'renders visible and public parts of our lives which previously remained hidden and offers them up to scrutiny' (Thorogood, 1992: 49).

In so far as it is experienced as a form of social control, health promotion prompts resistance. For instance, a community cancer education project that was intended to change the behaviour of white working class Americans was rejected through the use of a counter-discourse of fate (Balshem, 1991). This 'fatalism' was a form of community resistance to scientists' definition of their problems. Likewise, Bloor and McIntosh (1990) have documented how health visitors' surveillance of mothers can provoke various forms of resistance.

Health promotion, however, is interpreted very differently according to who delivers it and what their motives are perceived to be. There is a clear contrast, for instance, between the way gay men are likely to respond to gay AIDS activists promoting safer sex and heterosexuals' responses to government HIV education campaigns. In the former case:

> The self-conscious leadership and participation of gay men, as opposed to biomedical experts, in this endeavour suggests that individuals actively participate in creating and changing cultural and erotic meanings, particularly when they have a stake in doing so.
>
> (Vance, 1991:881)

For most British heterosexuals these conditions are reversed: their vulnerability to HIV has been asserted by biomedical scientists, and they have not actively participated in changing cultural and erotic meanings because the safer sex campaigns have been designed and imposed by such experts.

In order to assess whether the resistance to a particular campaign might outweigh its benefits, it is crucial to understand the cultural context of the behaviour one is trying to influence. One aspect of this context is the role that stage in the life course has in shaping what is considered reasonable behaviour with regard to health. Backett and Davison (1992) found that young single adults tend to view their bodies as resilient to health-damaging behaviours, and see having foresight about future health as boring and middle-aged. Such life stage-appropriate behaviour is probably particularly important in the area of sexuality where many people have a concept of a conventional sexual career in which having several partners precedes settling down.

In the mid-1980s there was considerable debate about how radical the HIV/AIDS campaign for heterosexuals should be (Homans and Aggleton, 1988). The outcome of considerable conflict within government departments (Miller and Williams, forthcoming) was a campaign that combined a moral message, to restrict partners/ be monogamous, with a less moralistic but still conservative one, use condoms.

Given the way in which safer sex was presented in the mass media it's not surprising that the young men in this sample assimilated the phrase into their pre-existing construction of sexuality. In particular, the primary meaning of sex was penetrative vaginal intercourse, and therefore safer sex excluded non-penetrative sex by definition. The homo-social context in which the men developed their sexuality made penetrative intercourse particularly significant, as a means of distinguishing virgins from non-virgins and demonstrating, or defining, the status of one's relationship with a woman. However, perhaps a clearer interpretation of what happened is that the young men did not assimilate a foreign health education message into their own culture, but rather, that the health education message came out of a heterosexual culture they already shared.

Despite the conservative approach to HIV health education there has been some resistance from heterosexuals, or at least institutions representing them. Its most obvious form is the collective ideological dissent of certain tabloid newspapers and the *Sunday Times* with their (continuing) campaign to belittle or deny the risk of HIV to heterosexuals (cf. Beharrell, 1993). Within my study one person actively disagreed with the HIV education campaign, a minority believed HIV was irrelevant to their lives and, for the rest, their main strategy to avoid infection was partner choice, not a change in sexual practices. Their understanding of the relative HIV risks of different sexual behaviours was largely irrelevant.

Many commentators have argued that a different approach to the HIV campaign for heterosexuals should have been adopted, one that challenged dominant heterosexual relations (see Homans and Aggleton, 1988; Wilton and Aggleton, 1991; Melia, 1989, Hart, 1993). In particular, presenting safer sex primarily as non-penetrative sex would contribute to deconstructing the equation of sex with penile penetration. Such a social transformatory approach

(Homans and Aggleton, 1988), it was argued, would empower women, educate the public about sexuality and eroticize relationships. The findings presented here offer some indication of the kind of resistance that such a radical approach from government bodies might have provoked.

Acknowledgements

Beyond the 58 young men who agreed to be interviewed in this study, I am particularly indebted to Sally Macintyre for her very constructive criticism of earlier drafts of this chapter. The work described is part of the MRC Medical Sociology Unit's programme and was funded by the Medical Research Council of Britain.

References

BACKETT, K. and DAVISON, C. (1992) 'Rational or reasonable? Perceptions of health at different stages of life', *Health Education Journal*, **51**, 2, pp. 55–9.

BALSHEM, M. (1991) 'Cancer, control and causality: Talking about cancer in a working-class community', *American Ethnologist*, **18**, 1, pp. 152–72.

BEHARRELL, P. (1993) 'AIDS and the British Press', in Glasgow University Media Group (Eds) *Getting the Message: News, Truth and Power*, London: Routledge.

BLOOR, M. and MCINTOSH, J. (1990) 'Surveillance and concealment: A comparison of techniques of client resistance in therapeutic communities and health visiting', in CUNNINGHAM-BURLEY, S. and MCKEGANEY, N. (Eds) *Readings in Medical Sociology*, London: Tavistock/Routledge.

BLOOR, M., ELDRIDGE, J., MACINTYRE, S., PHILO, G., BEHARRELL, P., KITZINGER, J., MILLER, D. and WILLIAMS, K. (1991) 'Sociological study of the content of AIDS media messages and audience responses', End of Award Report to the ESRC.

BUNTON, Robin (1992) 'More than a woolly jumper: health promotion as social regulation', *Critical Public Health*, **3**, 2, pp. 4–11.

DAVIES, S. (1991) *The Historical Origins of Health Fascism*, London: Forest.

FORD, N. (1991) 'The socio-sexual lifestyles of young people in the South West of England', Bristol: South Western Regional Health Authority.

HART, G. (1993) Safer sex: A paradigm revisited, in AGGLETON, P., DAVIES, P. and HART, G. (Eds) *AIDS: Facing the Second Decade*, London: Falmer Press.

HEALTH EDUCATION AUTHORITY/MORI (1990) 'Young adults' health and lifestyle: Sexual behaviour', London: Health Education Authority.

HOLLAND, J., RAMAZANOGLU, C., SCOTT, S., SHARPE, S. and THOMSON, R. (1991) 'Between embarrassment and trust: Young women and the diversity of condom use', in AGGLETON, P., DAVIES, P. and HART, G. (eds) *AIDS: Responses, Intervention and Care*, London: Falmer Press.

HOMANS, H. and AGGLETON, P. (1988) 'Health education, HIV infection and AIDS', in AGGLETON, P. and HOMANS, H. (Eds) *Social Aspects of AIDS*, Lewes: Falmer Press.

JOHNSON, A.M., WADSWORTH, J., WELLINGS, K. and FIELD, J. (1994) 'Sexual Attitudes and lifestyles', London: Blackwell Scientific.

KENT, V., DAVIES, M., DEVERELL, K. and GOTTESMAN, S. (1990) 'Social interaction routines involved in heterosexual encounters: prelude to first intercourse', paper presented at the Fourth Conference on Social Aspects of AIDS, South Bank Polytechnic, London, 7 April.

KITZINGER, J. (1993) 'Safer Sex and Dangerous Reputations: Contradictions for Young Women negotiating Condom Use', Working Paper No. 47, MRC Medical Sociology Unit, 6 Lilybank Gardens, Glasgow G12.

MACINTYRE, S. and WEST, P. (1993) 'What does the phrase safer sex mean to you?' Understandings among Glaswegian 18-year-olds in 1990, *AIDS* 7, pp. 121–125.

MCEWAN, R. and BHOPAL, R. (1991) *HIV/AIDS Health Promotion for Young People: A Review of Theory, Principles and Practice*, London: Health Education Authority.

MELIA, J. (1989) 'Sex education in schools: keeping to the norm', in JONES C. and MAHONEY, P. (Eds) *Learning our Lines, Sexuality and Sexual Control in Education*, London: The Women's Press.

MILLER, D. and BEHARRELL, P. (1993) 'AIDS and access to television: How journalists use their sources', paper presented to the British Sociological Association Annual Conference, Essex University, 5–8 April 1993.

MILLER, D. and WILLIAMS, K. (1993) 'Negotiating HIV/AIDS information: Agendas, media strategies and the news', in Glasgow University Media Group (Eds) *Getting the Message: News, Truth and Power*, London: Routledge.

MILLER, D. and WILLIAMS, K. (forthcoming) 'From icebergs and tombstones to personal testimony: The AIDS public education campaign, 1986–90', in Glasgow University Media Group (Eds) *Dying of Ignorance? AIDS, the Media and Public Beliefs*, London: Sage.

ROCHERON, Y. and LINNE, O. (1989) 'AIDS, moral panic and opinion polls', *European Journal of Communication*, 4, pp. 409–34.

SPENCER, B. (1984) 'Young men: their attitudes towards sexuality and birth control', *British Journal of Family Planning*, 10, pp. 13–19.

SPENCER, L., FAULKNER, A. and KEEGAN, J. (1988) *Talking About Sex: Asking the Public About Sexual Behaviour and Attitudes*, London: Social and Community Planning Research.

THOROGOOD, N. (1992) 'Sex education as social control', *Critical Public Health*, 3, 4, pp. 43–50.

VANCE, C.S. (1991) 'Anthropology rediscovers sexuality: A theoretical comment', *Social Science and Medicine*, 33, 8, pp. 875–84.

WHITE, D.G., PHILLIPS, K.C., PITTS, M., CLIFFORD, B.R., ELLIOT, J.R. and DAVIES, M.M. (1988) 'Adolescents' perceptions of AIDS', *Health Education Journal*, 47, 4, pp. 117–19.

WIGHT, D. (1993a) 'A re-assessment of health education on HIV/AIDS for young heterosexuals', *Health Education Research: Theory and Practice*, 8, 4, pp. 473–83.

WIGHT, D. (1993b) 'Constraint or cognition? Young men and safer heterosexual sex', in AGGLETON, P., DAVIES, P. and HART, G. (Eds) *AIDS: Facing the Second Decade*, London: Falmer Press.

WIGHT, D. (in press) 'Boys' thoughts and talk about sex in a working class locality of Glasgow', *Sociological Review*, forthcoming.

WILTON, T. and AGGLETON, P. (1991) 'Condoms, coercion and control: Heterosexuality and the limits to HIV/AIDS education', in AGGLETON, P., DAVIES, P. and HART, G. (Eds) AIDS: *Responses, Intervention and Care*, London: Falmer Press.

Chapter 8

Marital Discourse and Condom Use

Carla Willig

Despite relative media silence in recent months, new cases of HIV infection are still occurring in Britain as elsewhere in Europe. The rate of infection through heterosexual contact is increasing steadily. A record number of AIDS cases were reported by the Public Health Laboratory Service for the third quarter of 1992: a total of 417 new cases, which is more than the previously worst quarter (391 to the end of December 1991). Of these cases 216 have been attributed to heterosexual sex. It has been suggested that heterosexual behaviour shows little sign of change in order to cut the risk of HIV infection. According to Adler (1992) one in 100 men at London's STD clinics and one in 200 women at central London antenatal clinics are HIV positive. Whereas in 1987 heterosexual intercourse was responsible for 9 per cent of HIV infections, it was responsible for 30 per cent of infections in the first six months of 1993. There is also evidence that a large proportion of heterosexually active young people fail to use condoms regularly (e.g. Richard and van der Pligt, 1991; Ford, 1991; Ingham, Woodcock and Stenner 1991).

A number of approaches can be taken in order to explore people's reluctance to follow safer sex guidelines. The approach most popular among psychologists is to make use of existing behaviour models such as the Health Belief Model (Rosenstock, 1974; Becker, 1974) or the Theory of Reasoned Action (Fishbein and Ajzen, 1975). The latter has been used by a number of researchers in order to investigate young people's condom use (see Richard and van der Pligt, 1991; Rise, 1992). The theory has been found wanting in that it fails to incorporate relevant factors such as past behaviour, type of relationship and self-efficacy. In addition, Ingham *et al.* (1991, 1992; Willig, 1992) have criticized psychological models of health behaviour on the basis of their inherent rationalism. In their study of 95 young people's accounts of their first-ever intercourse, Ingham *et al.* (1991) identified three major reasons given for first intercourse. Among these were 'situational pressures' including 'uncontrollable urges' (usually physical), and being 'carried away' (usually emotional). Such 'irrational' or non-cognitive factors cannot easily be incorporated into rationalistic decision-making models. Maticka-Tyndale (1992) criticizes mainstream AIDS research for failing to address AIDS prevention strategies as personally constructed through common sense knowledge about AIDS. She draws attention to the relevance of social constructionist approaches to understanding the actions of young people potentially at risk of HIV infection.

In contrast to such models, discourse analytic approaches move beyond attempts to measure relevant variables and look at the social construction of meaning itself. Instead of using researcher-defined variables in order to predict health behaviour, discourse analysis aims to understand how people make sense of events. The focus is upon the discourses that are available to individuals, and moves away from what Henriques *et al.* (1984) have referred to as the *rational unitary subject*. For example, in order to better understand why people do or do not use condoms, we need to become aware of what these behaviours mean to participants. Holland *et al.*'s (1991) work with young women in London and Manchester investigating the negotiation of safer sex has revealed that condoms carry symbolic meanings. A woman's request for condom use, for example, constitutes a challenge to dominant constructions of heterosexual activity. 'When a young woman insists on the use of a condom for her own safety, she is going against the construction of sexual intercourse as man's natural pleasure and woman's natural duty' (Holland, *et al.*, 1991:131).

Holland *et al.*'s work reveals that young women's conceptualization of sex in terms of love, romance and relationships with men informed their choice of sexual practices, including penetrative sex and a reluctance to use condoms. Using a similar approach, Ingham *et al.* (1992) observed that a social construction of sexual activity as something mystical and uncontrollable allows people to justify and accept unsafe sexual behaviour as natural. After all, safer sex is not easily compatible with widespread notions of passion which are characterized by loss of control. A sexual encounter which requires planning and negotiation is easily perceived as premeditated and is not usually associated with love and passion.

The study reported here used discourse analysis in order better to understand heterosexual adults' accounts of condom use. Discursive constructions of what it means to use a condom in a relationship may constrain or facilitate particular behaviours within particular contexts. Warwick and Aggleton (1990:89) draw attention to the fact that the heterosexual adolescent, constructed by popular myths as 'deficient, irresponsible and developmentally immature' and therefore inherently at risk, has become the subject of numerous studies in the field of HIV and AIDS (along with other marginalized groups such as gay men, injecting drug users and sex workers). It was felt that it was time to focus on heterosexual adults, often constructed by the media as the general population, their positioning within AIDS-relevant discourses and their consequent vulnerability to HIV infection.

Analysing talk

The material presented in this chapter is drawn from a series of semi-structured interviews with 14 individuals, with equal numbers of males and females, and equal numbers of working class and middle class employees. Respondents were interviewed individually, and each interview lasted approximately one hour. The interview agenda included questions about the nature of HIV disease, its social and political implications as well as the respondent's personal feelings about HIV and AIDS. All interviews were tape-recorded and transcribed. All respondents had been contacted via their common employer and all had volunteered to participate.

This chapter discusses respondents' accounts of their own condom use. Parker's (1992:5) definition of discourse as 'a system of statements which constructs an object' was adopted. Consequently the aim of the analysis was to identify discourses which informed talk about condom use. Thus, rather than presenting subjects with a researcher-defined attitude object (i.e. condoms) in order to measure their attitudes towards it, the aim of this discourse analysis was to understand the ways in which respondents themselves construct the object. Discursive meanings are, therefore, *not* attitudes towards or even beliefs about, the object. Instead, discursive meanings actually construct the object itself. The analysis of interview data was guided by Parker's (1992:6) initial three 'steps in an analysis of discourse dynamics'. In order to identify relevant discourses, all references to condoms or condom use were identified and highlighted in the transcripts (*step one*: selection of text for analysis). The quotations were then organised thematically. Here, Strauss's (1987) grounded theory approach to categorization was adopted. This meant that themes emerged from the text, and that re-categorization of quotations took place throughout the analysis as new themes emerged. Quotations could be placed in more than one category and quotations could (and often did) embrace more than one theme. Organization by theme in this analysis fulfilled a similar function to *step two* in Parker's (1992:7) guide to the analysis of discourse, which requires 'a process of exploring the connotations, allusions and implications which the texts evoke'. This was followed by an exploration of the ways in which the object (i.e. condom use) is constructed in the texts (*step three*). A close examination of respondents' construction of sets of meanings defining the object led to the identification of a dominant discourse.

Constituting the discourse

Respondents framed their accounts of condom use almost exclusively within a marital discourse. This discourse constructs marriage as a condition incompatible with condom use. Furthermore, respondents' assumptions regarding the nature of marriage, as safe by definition and based upon trust, together with their belief that relationships can 'go wrong', position married respondents in such a way that they feel unable to request safer sex from their spouse. The remainder of this section will trace some of the ways in which these major elements of a marital discourse are constituted.

Assumptions of Safety

Respondents established an association between marriage and safety whereby being married came to signify a state of safety with regard to HIV. Such an association was expressed in two different ways. First, a reference to a person's marital status was presented as *sufficient grounds* for an assumption of safety and/or immunity in relation to the possibility of HIV infection. Second, it was suggested that spouses are *required* to trust each other and are therefore *obliged* to assume that they are safe. For example, Ian argues:

> Somebody who marries, for example, and trusts their partner but their partner is HIV positive and hasn't told them, then they're an innocent victim too, because again relationships are built on trust and maybe they asked their partner as it would be indeed prudent to do. If their partner said no, I'm clear, then they *would have* to believe it. (my emphasis).

Assumptions of safety were not restricted to married couples. Respondents tended to include steady relationships, or what is often referred to as 'long-term, stable relationships', in their marital discourse. For example, Tina said she used condoms with someone she 'had a bit of an affair with', but not with Reg, her steady partner. She assumes safety with the latter. Tom's definition of innocent victims includes both a husband and a wife as well as 'poor unsuspecting girlfriends and boyfriends', again suggesting that a steady relationship is equivalent to a marriage with regard to sexual safety. However, Tom's example of those who are 'in between' guilty and innocent with regard to HIV infection describes a scenario of impulsive sex involving a girlfriend or boyfriend who gets carried away at a party and has sexual intercourse outside the relationship. The fact that there are no husbands or wives in this scenario suggests that according to Tom there are stages towards safety, with marriage representing the highest stage. The following comment made by Tom further specifies the parameters of such a hierarchy of safety. Tom feels no need to use condoms, because of the long duration of his marriage (36 years) and the nature of his relationship ('happy' and 'old fashioned'). In his construction of a safe relationship, age is crucial: young people are not safe whatever their relationships. 'Old-fashioned couples who've been married for many, many years' are safe, whereas young couples have a problem: 'these days most young people getting married, are getting married after they've had sex anyway, so again the stable door is shut after the horse has bolted' (Tom). Thus, respondents tend to make their attributions of safety on the basis of category membership such as marital status and age, rather than by reference to individual characteristics and behaviours.

Attributions of safety were occasionally made following a disclaimer. For example, Lee at one and the same time acknowledges that marriage is no guarantee for safety, yet she accounts for her friends' safety by reference to their marital status. When asked whether she worries about her friends with regard to the possibility of HIV infection, she responds:

> No, because I think unfortunately most of us are all boring and all married (laughs), *not, not for that reason, of course, ah, that's no protection*, I think most of them are sort of in pretty stable marriages, where as far, *although of course you can never vouch for their partners*, their husband or wife, um, but as far as I can tell they're sort of staying very loyal to each other, um, no, I haven't got any worries about my friends. (my emphasis)
>
> (Lee)

A disclaimer, defined by Hewitt and Stokes (1975) as a verbal device which is used to ward off potentially negative attributions, functions by acknowledging a possible interpretation while denying it at the same time. In this case Lee disclaims the attribution that she has not understood the latest AIDS education message that 'anyone can be infected thus everyone is at risk ('. . . not for that reason, of course, that's no protection . . .') but denies its applicability to her friends and to herself ('*We* are all boring and all married . . .' my emphasis). Lee's use of this disclaimer is particularly interesting when we consider the fact that Lee is not married herself.

The assumption that marriage is safe structured respondents' comments about bachelorship. For respondents, sexual vulnerability was associated with the single status. For Pete, the 'modern lifestyle' involves being single, unattached or not permanently attached, not with any great commitments and it makes people more susceptible to HIV infection. According to Sam, there are 'vulnerable groups' characterized by unstable lifestyles and a less than normal environment which can be contrasted with family life. Tina says she would have an HIV antibody test 'if I became single again', but not now that she is with Reg. This implies that the single status *per se* is unsafe, even though being single might mean not having sexual intercourse at all, whereas her relationship with Reg definitely involves sexual activity.

Many accounts based on the marital discourse establish an association between 'settled safety' and age. Marriage, and its near equivalent (the long-term, stable relationship) are constructed as a safe haven which people eventually reach as they mature. Tom justifies his concern about the vulnerability of his sons to HIV with a reference to their marital status, and at the same time assumes that eventually they will be married and therefore safe: he worries because he has 'sons neither of whom are married *yet* . . .' (my emphasis). Similarly, when talking about his anxieties about his teenage sons, Jon identifies a 'high-risk slot' related to age and marital status which is located between school and marriage. Both these institutions are perceived to protect the individual. Again, however, such constructions of 'settled safety' are not restricted to the married relationship. Tina suggests that the older one gets, the more one tends to stick with one partner. Again, the notion of settling down is associated with safety. Tina explains, 'But I think as you get older, people sort of tend to settle down with one partner for a while, don't they, and I think as you get older, you probably tend to stick with one partner.'

Here, it is suggested that it is a natural development that people eventually find a safe haven characterized by stability and monogamy. However, the notion of safety as a function of something settled extends to even less traditional relationships: Anne's account of why she does not practice safer sex revolves around her sense of security due to her knowledge of her sexual partner and his sexual partner(s) due to 'settled situations'. When asked why she does not use condoms, she says:

> Well, because you think to yourself, you think you know the other person's sexual behaviour, and you think even if you know they're having sex with more than just you, you think you know who else they're having sex with, and you think that's only two . . . so you think, oh sod it. You know you think I suppose you mean, if you do bother to think, you think, ah well, the odds are that with only two or, two, say, two sexual partners or something that the odds are that, it'll be alright . . . *particularly if you know all the situations are very settled*, you don't, but I think probably if you were younger and, um, I would probably be more careful . . . (my emphasis).
>
> (Anne)

Again, it is not specific activities but the categories of stable relationship(s) and age that are associated with safety. The categories that constitute marital discourse enable Anne to assume sexual safety for herself: to be a mature woman who is involved in settled relationships is to be safe.

Assumptions of Trust

Trust was identified by respondents as a crucial defining feature of marriage. Respondents' accounts typically revolved around the notion of trust. Trust was called upon to justify a reluctance to use condoms. This was done either by arguing that the existing trust in the relationship made it unnecessary to use condoms or, much more frequently (and much more interestingly), by suggesting that the request to use a condom would undermine trust and thus damage the relationship.

For example, Jane points out that she does not use condoms because she trusts her husband and that she 'wouldn't have married the guy if I'd had to do that'. Here, the notion of trust is called upon in order to justify the decision not to use condoms. The existing trust in the relationship makes condom use unnecessary. However, respondents acknowledge that trust needs to be re-established all the time, and that it is vulnerable to being undermined. Thus, trust is perceived not as a stable attribute of a relationship but rather as an interactive process. It is seen as something which is continuously re-created out of two people's behaviour towards one another. Within this context, the suggestion to use a condom within a trusting relationship constitutes a threat to the assumption of safety which characterizes marriage. For example, Sam points out that his marriage is based on trust. He explains that the use of condoms would constitute an insult to his marriage and to his wife, and that,

> It wouldn't do that relationship any good at all if some sort of doubt was injected into it by suggesting that possibly one of us could be having an affair and to be absolutely certain we must use a condom.
>
> (Sam)

Sam has been married for 30 years, the last 10 to 15 of which have been monogamous. The trust that has been established between Sam and his wife since the marriage became monogamous could easily be undermined by the suggestion that there is no guarantee for monogamy at the present time. The maintenance of trust requires that the assumption of sexual safety is not questioned either behaviourally or verbally.

Sue provides a very clear account of the dynamics of trust when she talks about the history of her marriage. She explains that she would hesitate to suggest condom use to her partner, even though it would be a 'sensible way to behave', because, '. . . after some difficulties we have built up a very considerable degree of trust in each other, and I wouldn't want to do anything that would start to remove that' (Sue). In other words, the sensible way to behave is not always conducive to the maintenance of trust. When asked about the difficulties preceding the establishment of trust, Sue explains that her husband's last extramarital affair, three or four years ago caused a 'big, big shake-up in our life' leading to the decision to have a child. Sue and her partner did not talk about the risk of HIV infection ('And I didn't actually say anything to him about it, neither of us ever, ever talked about it in terms of ourselves'), but Sue felt that the fact that her husband was willing to conceive with her indicated that he believed himself not to be infected: 'I felt pretty sure that if he felt there was any sort of danger, then he wouldn't have attempted to conceive with me, and I suppose that was the thing that really turned the (tables) for me . . .' (Sue).

Sue's account indicates that the establishment of trust required careful manipulation of symbols. Her husband's preparedness to conceive a child signalled to Sue that he was safe. Thus, his commitment to having a child carries a number of meanings for Sue, one of which signifies sexual safety. Hollway (1989), in her analysis of two women's accounts of becoming pregnant, identified a similar association between making love without contraception and securing commitment to a relationship. Here, the relationship between the two terms is established through a third term, 'having a baby'. Hollway conceptualizes this as an instance of metonymy, i.e. the movement of meaning from one signifier to another where due to their firm connection making love without contraception and having a baby both come to signify securing commitment.

In addition, for Sue, the continuation of trust meant *not* raising challenging questions. '. . . and since that time, I haven't wanted to rock the boat, and it's the same reasons why now I couldn't go to him and say, why don't we wear condoms forever and ever (laughs)' (Sue). Here, the need to preserve trust is associated with marital insecurity and a sense of fragility. Sue is careful not to 'rock the boat'. Again, as for Sam, trust had to be built up over a period of time, and its maintenance requires strict control over what is and what is not said. And again, trust is extremely important to the relationship precisely because the latter is so vulnerable due to its history.

It appears, then, that *not* talking about things and *not* asking certain questions, is much more fundamental to the development and maintenance of a trusting relationship than to talk honestly and openly. Respondents' understanding of the notion of trust is therefore very different from that promoted by AIDS education materials where trusting your partner means being able to talk with your partner about your sexual relationship and where trust is portrayed as a facilitator of communication. It does not take on this meaning for respondents. The opposite appears to be the case. Respondents seem to feel that there is only a need to talk when things are going wrong. For example, Jane acknowledges that the nature of her relationship based on trust and safety could change and that there is no guarantee for safety. After she has pointed out that she trusts her husband while acknowledging that 'there's nobody who can ever be sure that their partner is being entirely faithful, you've just got to trust them', Jane speculates about the future:

> At the moment I feel like the future is pretty safe. How long have we been married, what, six months, so everything is sort of rosy and everything. I dunno, um, I think if things started to change we'd probably have to do some talking.
>
> (Jane)

Thus, from within a marital discourse partners only need to talk about their sexual practices when problems arise. Consequently, the suggestion to talk may indicate to one's partner that something must indeed be wrong. Consequently, raising the issue of condom use with one's partner may well constitute a serious threat to the integrity of the relationship itself.

Assumptions of Possible Marital Failure

Respondents also acknowledged that the nature of a relationship can change. Being married requires trusting one's spouse (with one's life, in the context of HIV infection) but at the same time, there is no guarantee of safety. For example, Pete suggests that marriages can go wrong and not be as they should be, causing one of the partners to stray. Thus, marriage is no guarantee for safety. The notion of risk enters into the concept of marriage itself: if marriages can go wrong or fail, spouses will need particular skills to make them work. A marriage constitutes an achievement by two people. Sam illustrates this by drawing attention to the vulnerability of marital relationships:

> . . . because its a very tricky thing, there's pride and there's suspicion and there's jealousy, and there's all these terrible things all mixed up together, and these are the things that kill a marriage, and therefore it's a very delicate ground that you're treading on.
>
> (Sam)

Accounts such as this suggest that respondents perceive marriages as finely balanced, delicate creatures that need to be nurtured and looked after. They are permanently under threat from undermining influences such as Sam's jealousy, pride and suspicion or Lee's mad flings and temptation: 'You can't afford to be complacent, I mean, just because you are a happily married man or a happily married woman category, that the fact that one day they might be tempted to have a fling, that the consequences could be this' (Lee). This discourse acknowledges that relationships, including marriage, can go wrong. There is no guarantee that a marriage will be as it should be. The two people involved need to make the relationship work, and this can fail. This discourse, therefore, constructs marriage, and its equivalents, as fragile, carefully balanced creations, which require effort and sensitivity to be made to work. It is also assumed that there is an ideal state of marriage, characterized by monogamy, to which all marriages aspire. Marriages which do not conform to the ideal constitute failures. It follows that even in marriage there is no guarantee for safety.

Marital discourse and its applicationss

This analysis of people's accounts of condom use has identified a widely used discourse which may help us understand many couples' reluctance to use condoms. Marital discourse constructs marriage (and its equivalents) as a relationship which is based upon trust and which generates safety. Within this discourse, assumptions of safety are not only justified but required. This is because the trust which characterizes marriage needs to be maintained and re-established constantly. Consequently, any suggestion that an assumption of safety may not be entirely justified constitutes a challenge to the basis of the relationship. It follows that far from the popular claim that married couples need not use condoms, we have a situation where married couples *cannot afford* to use condoms. And involvement in a trusting relationship is not necessarily a protection against HIV infection as suggested by health education materials, instead it may operate as a barrier against communication with one's partner. Certain topics many not be broached because their mention would undermine trust. The suggestion to use condoms constitutes a powerful threat to the fragile behavioural balancing act that makes a marriage. The acknowledgement that relationships can change, that there is no guarantee for a happy marriage and that a marriage must be made to work by its participants is fundamental to the discourse. The belief that marriage *ought* to be safe, combined with the belief that marriage *can* fail, requires the setting up of trust as the crucial mediator. In order to demonstrate the existence of trust, couples must *assume* safety. In order for a marriage to work, spouses must behave as though there was a guarantee for safety, precisely because there is none. These findings have behavioural implications. Marital discourse positions the married individual in such a way that s/he is unable to request safer sex. The discourse disempowers its users, and at the present time makes them vulnerable to HIV infection.[1] The risk is increased by the fact that, as we have seen, marital discourse is also used by those who *perceive* themselves to be in steady relationships, including serial monogamy and multiple partners. Such 'importing' of marital discourse may have direct implications for sexual behaviour. The observation that adolescents tend to use condoms at first intercourse and/or with irregular partners, but stop or switch to other forms of contraceptions once relationships are formed (e.g. Richard and van der Pligt, 1991), may be indicative of the normative powers of marital discourse. Supporting such a line of thought, in her analysis of 25 in-depth interviews with Canadian college students, Maticka-Tyndale (1992) identified reliance on trust as a method of protection against HIV infection. Women in particular found themselves unable to request condom use from partners whom they knew well. As with the respondents here, their conceptualization of trust meant that 'they were most able to protect themselves from . . . pregnancy, disease and emotional hurt in casual sexual encounters' (Maticka-Tyndale, 1992: 247) because introducing condoms was perceived to violate the trust on which 'serious' relationships are based. Interestingly, Maticka-Tyndale's analysis revealed a gender difference in respondents' conceptualizations of trust which was not identified in this study. Future analyses of the role of trust in the negotiation of safer sex need to be sensitive to possible gender differences in respondents' constructions of trust.

In this chapter the focus has been upon a particular discourse and its employment in respondents' talk about condom use. However, little attention has been paid to the function of the discourse. If we adopt Potter and Wetherell's (1987) conceptualization of discourse as social action we may speculate that the use of marital discourse in the context of HIV and AIDS allows respondents to self-categorize as safe. It is quite possible that in another context, such as when talking to friends about recent holidays, respondents' accounts may be framed by other discourses with different functions, for example, to portray oneself as 'good time girl' or 'one of the lads'.[2] It is, however impossible to establish the function of marital discourse in this investigation since, as suggested by Gilbert and Mulkay (1984), in order to do this we would need to study variability in the way that the object is constructed across contexts.

A further dimension of discourse analysis which requires additional attention is the grounding of the discourse in social reality (see Parker, 1992, Chapter 2). It could be argued that marital discourse is grounded in the social institution of the nuclear family which is often portrayed as the fundamental unit of society. According to Barrett and McIntosh (1991) marriage is 'massively privileged by social policy, taxation, religious endorsement and the accolade of respectability' (ibid.:56) in order to promote the nuclear family. Marital discourse can be understood as one dimension of what Barrett and McIntosh call *familialism*, i.e. 'ideologies modelled on what are thought to be family values' (ibid.:26). More work is needed in order to explore the ways in which marital discourse overlaps and interacts with familial discourse, and to investigate their historical origins.

To conclude, a focus on the discursive construction of objects and an understanding of what it is possible to say at a particular moment provides a helpful framework for looking at marital discourse as a discourse with normative powers in the context of HIV infection. The identification of marital discourse in respondents' talk about condom use has contributed to our understanding of why it is that both married and unmarried couples are reluctant to request condom use from their partners.

Notes

1 The extent of people's vulnerability is highlighted when we consider that 30 per cent of marriages end in divorce, as well as recent evidence which suggests that 50 per cent of young men engaged to be married were unfaithful with two or more women when on holiday without their fiancées (Ford, 1991).
2 Hollway (1989) identifies a 'discourse of male sex drive' whose central proposition is that men are driven by the biological necessity to seek out (heterosexual) sex. Hollway suggests that this discourse is widely used in a variety of contexts, both institutional, for example, male judges' tendency to impose lenient sentences on rapists and

personal, for example, men trying to make sense of their experience of their own sexuality. It is possible that male respondents' accounts of a recent holiday or a party may be framed by the 'discourse of male sexual drive', where this positions the respondent as a 'proper man', rather than by marital discourse which position the respondent as safe.

Acknowledgement

I would like to thank Kathryn Lovering and Timothy Auburn for making helpful comments on an earlier draft of this paper.

References

ADLER, M. (1992) 'Sexual trends "point to AIDS epidemic for heterosexuals",' *The Guardian*, 12th November, p. 3.

BARRETT, M. and MCINTOSH, M. (1991) *The Antisocial Family*, London: Verso.

BECKER, M. (1974) *The Health Belief Model and Personal Health Behaviour*, Thorofare, NJ: Charles B. Slack.

FISHBEIN, M. and AJZEN, I. (1975) *Belief, Attitude and Behaviour: An Introduction to Theory and Research*, Reading, MA: Addison-Wesley.

FORD, N. (1991) 'Sex on Holiday: The HIV-Related Sexual Interaction of Young Tourists Visiting Torbay', *Occasional Working Paper No. 14*, Institute of Population Studies, University of Essex.

GILBERT, N. and MULKAY, M. (1984) *Opening Pandora's Box: A Sociological Analysis of Scientists' Discourse*, Cambridge: Cambridge University Press.

HENRIQUES, J., HOLLWAY, W., URWIN, C., VENN, C. and WALKERDINE, V. (1984) *Changing the Subject: Psychology, Social Relations and Subjectivity*, London: Methuen.

HEWITT, J.P. and STOKES, R. (1975) 'Disclaimers', *American Sociological Review*, **40**, pp. 1–11.

HOLLAND, J., RAMAZANOGLU, C., SCOTT, S., SHARPE, S. and THOMSON, R. (1991) 'Between embarrassment and trust: Young women and the diversity of condom use', in AGGLETON, P., HART, G. and DAVIES, P. (Eds) *AIDS: Responses, Interventions and Care*, London: Falmer Press.

HOLLWAY, W. (1989) *Subjectivity and Method in Psychology*, London: Sage.

INGHAM, R., WOODCOCK, A. and STENNER, K. (1991) 'Getting to know you . . . young people's knowledge of their partners at first intercourse', *Journal of Community and Applied Social Psychology*, **1**, 2, pp. 117–32.

INGHAM, R., WOODCOCK, A. and STENNER, K. (1992) 'The limitations of rational decision-making models as applied to young people's sexual behaviour', in AGGLETON, P., DAVIES, P. and HART, G. (Eds) *AIDS, Rights, Risk and Reason*, London: Falmer Press.'

MATICKA-TYNDALE, E. (1992) 'Social construction of HIV transmission and prevention among young heterosexual adults', *Social Problems*, **39**, 3.

PARKER, I. (1992) *Discourse Dynamics. Critical Analysis for Social and Individual Psychology*, London: Routledge.

Carla Willig

POTTER, J. and WETHERELL, M. (1987) *Discourse and Social Psychology*, London: Sage.

RICHARD, R. and VAN DER PLIGT, J. (1991) 'Factors affecting condom use among adolescents', *Journal of Community and Applied Social Psychology*, 1, pp. 105–16.

RISE, J. (1992) 'An empirical study of the decision to use condoms among Norwegian adolescents using the theory of reasoned action', *Journal of Community and Applied Social Psychology*, 2, 3, pp. 185–97.

ROSENSTOCK, I.M. (1974) 'Historical origins of the health belief model', *Health Education Monographs*, 2, pp. 328–35.

STRAUSS, A. (1987) *Qualitative Analysis for Social Scientists*, Cambridge: Cambridge University Press.

WARWICK, I. and AGGLETON, P. (1990) '"Adolescents", young people and AIDS research', in AGGLETON, P., DAVIES, P. and HART, G. (Eds) *AIDS: Individual, Cultural and Policy Dimensions*, Basingstoke: Falmer Press.

WILLIG, C. (1992) 'Assumptions in people's talk about AIDS', *Journal of Community and Applied Social Psychology*, 2, 3, pp. 217–21.

Chapter 9

Sexual Exchange: Understanding Pre-marital Heterosexual Relationships in Urban Ghana

Augustine Ankomah and Nicholas Ford

A review of the pre- and post-AIDS literature on sexual life in Africa reveals numerous research approaches and interpretations which are basically western in the implicit assumptions they make, and which are therefore unlikely to enhance the effectiveness of HIV-related intervention strategies. There is a pressing need for research into sexual behaviour in particular cultural contexts to provide some understanding of the prevailing sexual life so as to contribute towards the development of potentially effective HIV prevention strategies. There were 145 cases of AIDS in Ghana by February 1988. The number had increased to 590 in April 1989, with 85 per cent of reported cases being females. As at 1 January 1993 there were 8345 reported HIV seropositives out of which 67 per cent were women (Ministry of Health, 1993).

The relatively few pre-AIDS anthropological studies (Little, 1973; Bleek, 1976; Pellow, 1977) provide some insight into the socio cultural context of sex in Ghana. While not every sexual relationship of single women in the urban centres of Ghana involves payment or the receipt of gifts or favours, sexual service tend to be regarded as something which is obtained by favour or by bargaining, a practice quite different from prostitution in the classic western sense. Pecuniary interest may, in an expediency, take precedence over the relationship itself. Economic pressures, among others, provide the background for most sexual relationships from which material gain is expected (Acquah, 1972; Assimeng, 1981; Dinan, 1983; Akuffo, 1987). Consequently, it is the nature, extent and the reasons behind this kind of sexual exchange rather than formal prostitution which demands attention of researchers seeking to better understand mainstream sexual culture in Ghana. The main objective of this chapter, therefore, is to explore within the socio-cultural and appropriate theoretical contexts the key factors that explain sexual behaviour with particular reference to the nature of pre-marital relationships and partner change. Condom use is however beyond the scope of this discussion.

Social Exchange Theory

Premarital sexual life in urban Ghana involves a series of exchanges. It is generally considered that women confer upon men a favour by agreeing to their sexual advances, not only to provide them sexual gratification but also as a means of enhancing the man's personal self-esteem. The men are expected in return to provide women with cash or other material support. Men and women are interested in entering and continuing premarital sexual relationships that are rewarding to them. These basic notions relate to social exchange theory and are applied in this chapter to premarital sexual relationships. Social exchange is conceived of as associations involving 'actions that are contingent on rewarding reactions from others and that cease when these expected reactions are not forthcoming' (Blau, 1964:6). Implied, therefore, is a two-sided, mutually contingent and mutually rewarding process involving transactions or exchange based on the assumption that a resource will continue to flow only if there is a valued return contingent upon it (Emerson, 1976; Chadwick-Jones, 1976).

Although exchange theory has been widely used in sociology (Emerson, 1976), the application of the exchange framework in intimate relations has been recent and generally unappealing to most researchers. Traditionally, most exchange theorists have concerned themselves with less intense relationships, such as friendship choices (Chadwick-Jones, 1979). Even researchers who believe that exchange principles can be successfully applied to sexual relationships seem ambivalent and shy away from viewing close relationships in terms of exchange (Rubin, 1973). As suggested by Huston and Cate (1979), the basic tenets of exchange theory seem contrary (at least outwardly) to the western view of the nature of love and intimacy. Love is supposed to involve 'caring, altruism, communion and selflessness' and hence the idea that 'love is anchored in the exchange of rewards seems crass from such a perspective' (Huston and Cate, 1979:263).

In Ghana, perhaps because of the acute imbalance of allocation of resources, sexual exchange is becoming increasingly popular as a means of transferring resources from men who monopolize most positions of influence and power and are also controllers of financial resources, to women whose opportunities are very limited. In the traditional society there were diverse patterns in sexual culture, but exchange in sexual relationships was hardly a feature (Ankomah, 1992a). The modern trend is towards greater sexual exchange, multiple sexual partnering and partner-switching. These are related to structural developments resulting from unequal access to power and resources by gender. Modernization, and with it increased urbanization and gradual shift of traditional subsistence economic systems into national and international consumerist systems have had a radical impact on sexual behaviour. Gender inequality in the traditional society has resulted in imbalances in educational and job opportunities in the modern sector. With very limited opportunities, the status of most women is generally linked to their relationship to men, usually through marriage, and it is in the sphere of sex that women's bargaining power can be primarily brought to bear. Material well-being is therefore relatively bound up with sexual lifestyle. The recession in the Ghanaian economy which began in the late 1970s has exacerbated the utilization of sexual relationships for material gain. Yet no systematic attempt has been made empirically to subject pre-marital sexual networking to analysis using the exchange framework. It is in this context that this study is relevant in understanding the exchange connotations within pre-marital relationships in the urban setting in Ghana.

Methods

In order to minimize the threats to validity of data on sexual behaviour and also to obtain detailed information to understand contemporary sexual life, the study employed a number of different methods: a quantitative survey, in-depth interviews and focus group discussions. A representative sample of 400 residents was selected from the population of single females aged 18–25 years residing in the urban centre of Cape Coast, Ghana. A three-stage stratified probability sampling design involving electoral areas, electoral wards, and finally houses, was employed to recruit respondents. The questionnaire included items which covered personal socio-demographic characteristics, knowledge about HIV and risk-reduction measures, sexual behaviour and attitude to material recompense for sex. A Likert-type scale was constructed to measure attitudes.

Interviewing was done by 10 female students after initial training. Interviews were conducted in respondents' homes and as far as possible were not within earshot of third parties. In addition, in-depth interviews involving 39 young single men and 39 young single women, and focus group discussions for both females and males (three groups of each) were used to obtain data on respondents' subjective experiences regarding the attitudinal questions. The quality of data in sex research especially in Africa is crucially important in view of the misgivings people have as to whether such a sensitive issue is 'researchable'. In this study attempts were made to minimize threats to validity. This by no means suggests that all biases have been controlled, a task quite impossible in social science research. However, all possible threats known either from the literature or from the researchers' own experience were anticipated and as far as possible all practical measures taken to reduce potential biases.

An overview of sexual behaviour

This section provides a brief summary of respondents' sexual behaviour based on three indicators: age at first sexual intercourse (defined as penile-vaginal

Table 9.1   Cumulative percentage of sexually experienced respondents 1991

Age at First Intercourse	Sexually experienced respondents n = 344 per cent	All respondents n = 400 per cent
15 and below	23	20
16	42	36
17	60	52
18	79	68
19	89	77
20	96	83
21	99	86
22	100	86
Virgins	0	14
TOTAL	100	100

Table 9.2   Current number of sexual partners of single women (18–25), Cape Coast, Ghana: 1991

Number of partners	All respondents n = 400		Sexually experienced n = 344	
	Total	per cent	Total	per cent
Virgins	56	14	–	–
0	40	10	40	12
1	216	54	216	63
2	73	18	73	21
3 or more	15	4	15	4
TOTAL	400	100	344	100

penetrative sex), current number of sexual partners, and duration of sexual relationships. *Sexual partner* refers to person with whom an individual has engaged in sexual intercourse, and *sexually experienced* means those who have ever engaged in sexual intercourse.

First, there is a high level of sexual experience. An overwhelming proportion of the 400 respondents (86 per cent) had engaged in sexual intercourse at least once. For this group of non-virgins, as can be seen in Table 9.1, the commencement of sexual activity was fairly early. Two out of every five (42 per cent) had engaged in sexual intercourse by the time they were aged 16 years. The median age at first sexual intercourse was 17 years, and by this age three out of every five non-virgins had had sexual intercourse. The majority (63 per cent) of sexually experienced respondents (54 per cent of the entire sample) had only one partner (Table 9.2).

Although serial monogamy appears to be the feature of most premarital sexual relationships, one-quarter of sexually experienced respondents had more than one sexual partner at the time of the survey. There is, however, substantive evidence of partner switching as many respondents preferred to break an economically non-viable relationship instead of taking on an additional partner. This is typified by the following respondent:

> I was seventeen years old when I had my first sexual intercourse. Since then my current partner is the fourth one. I broke with the first one because he liked women too much! The second one did not give me enough money to cater for my needs, so I 'snubbed' him (i.e. broke the relationship). The third one gave me a lot of money but had a very bad character. He beat me often, so I left him.
>
> (21-year-old female, Form 4 leaver, unemployed)

As a result of frequent partner switching, the median duration of sexual relationships is just over one year (13 months). Only half of non-virgins had been in their current relationships for more than one year. Half of sexually experienced respondents did not engage in sexual intercourse during the four-week period prior to the survey. Those who had did so only on one or two occasions. For many women intercourse usually takes place when she visits the man. Many women explained that they visited their boyfriends infrequently since they (the men) demanded intercourse during such visits. Similar to the observations of Orubuloye, Caldwell and Caldwell, (1991) in the Ekiti district of western Nigeria, current or continuing relationships do not necessarily have to be cemented by sexual intercourse each week, or even each month, to be regarded as relationships with some continuity. Coital frequency is lower among highly educated women, presumably because their education and status place them in a better position to rebuff their partners' demands for sex.

The riskiness of a woman's sexual behaviour is not adequately explained by personal and demographic characteristics. For example, the number of a woman's current number of sexual partners is not associated with education, religion, age, ethnic background, parity occupation or income. It can therefore be concluded that other factors inherent in the nature of the society appear to offer more convincing explanations.

Attitudes to material recompense for sex

The key theoretical underpinning of the discussion is that social exchange principles are intrinsically and extrinsically inherent in most pre-marital sexual relationships. Among the sample, to a very large extent, sexual relationships are characterized by consumerism. The young woman exacts an exchange: sex for material gain. Within this broad phenomenon of sexual exchange, three different aspects can be distinguished. These are first, general views on the inherent exchange and consumerism in premarital relationships; second, views on premarital 'partner-sharing' provided consumerism is unaffected; and third, views on partner switching to maintain consumerism.

General Views on Exchange Principles within Relationships

In most of urban Ghana the notion of exchange and the transactions that go with it in a pre-marital relationship are clear not only to both partners but the society at large (Ankomah, 1992a; Ankomah and Ford, 1993). The material gains which women expect from sexual relationships are not symbolic, as some anthropologists seem to imply (Befu, 1977), but have economic value. In fact, they constitute the very core of the relationship. It is the absence of material recompense rather than its presence which is considered abnormal. As a sequel most women consider it natural for a man to provide for his partners in relationships. A focus group participant stated with characteristic directness: 'I expect money and other things. After all what are relationships about then? Men are supposed to provide money and all other things needed. If you don't have money why do you take a girlfriend in the first place?' (20-year-old female; 'chop bar' attendant)

The view that sexual relationships are predominantly consumerist in nature is not held by women alone. Men are consciously aware of them too and a majority endorsed the phenomenon, although a minority detested it insisting that they had no girlfriends because they did not have any money. This view was rebuffed by others. A male respondent offered some advice to his friends while at the same time chastising those who renege on providing material recompense to girlfriends. 'Men must know that their girls eat and put on dresses and if you will not provide these, then whom do you expect to provide for the girl?' (23-year-old male, national service personnel). Blau (1964) in his 'excursus on love', emphasized women's lack of interest in the rewards they obtain in the exchange processes within relationships. He noted: 'a woman may encourage a man to give her things and to do things for her not primarily out of interest in the material benefits but in order to foster his love for her.' (Blau, 1964:78).

The findings discussed above are different from those of Blau and the few researchers who have applied the exchange framework in studying sexual relationships within western contexts. First, contrary to the view of some exchange theorists (see Befu, 1977) that the existence of money in exchange transaction is purely symbolic, the evidence from this study shows that money and other material gain form the basis of premarital sexual relationships. Second, both partners in the relationship are clearly aware of the transactions that go in the relationship. Thus, unlike in the United States where Scanzoni

(1972) and Scanzoni and Scanzoni (1976) suggested that partners may not be consciously aware of the exchange transactions that operate in the relationship, in this case both partners know of its existence and women pragmatically try to maintain the favourable terms of exchange. The relationship is constantly monitored and assessed, and logical and rational decisions are made in cases where there is a break in the flow of material again. It is to the attitudes of the respondents towards the pragmatic tactics used to maintain sexual exchange that attention now turns.

Premarital partner-sharing: traditionalist vs. revisionist viewpoints

Polygyny is generally acceptable in most of Ghana and according to the Ghana Demographic and Health Survey about a third of all married women are in polygynous union (Statistical Service, 1989). Similarly in premarital sexual relationships it is a common practice for a man to have multiple partners. Since two or more women sharing one man has direct epidemiological linkage in terms of HIV infection, woman were asked how they would respond to such a relationship within the exchange framework.

Nearly two-thirds (58 per cent) are willing to enter into a relationship as a co-partner provided the exchange transactions are considered favourable. The traditionalists argued that men will always philander and that even within marriage, Ghanaian men have always been allowed to have more than one partner, hence there is no need to complain at the pre-marital stage, especially if the consumerist nature of the relationship is unaffected. 'Nothing can be done'; 'They will always do it'; 'They can't change'; and 'Society allows them', are some of the standard women's responses to this double standard morality. The following instance, of the 'every man does it' approach characterizes the traditionalist viewpoint held by over half of the women interviewed. 'I don't care; after all he is a man. If he can provide the things I need, I don't have to worry.' (23-year-old female; orange seller). Women's fear of their partners' relationship with other women is hardly emotional; rather they fear being cheated out of material things. Many of those who asserted that they are not bothered by their boyfriends' infidelity said that this was conditional upon their being given things that they expect.

Sexual relationships devoid of material gain

The prevailing severe economic conditions in Ghana which affect men and women while exacerbating women's expectation of material gain from sexual exchange has in practice affected their actual gains. Most men simply renege on their due. For example while 55 per cent of sexually active respondents expected their boyfriends to provide them with capital to start trading, only 15 per cent had actually had their expectations met. Women faced with this rapidly increasing loss in sexual exchange relationships have two broad pragmatic responses. These can be classified as immediate exchange strategists and deferred exchange strategists.

Immediate Exchange Strategists

The survey data show that over two-thirds of the respondents saw nothing wrong in terminating a relationship in which material gains are not forthcoming. To them, as explained by some women in the qualitative interviews, instant material gains seem to override the possibility of any future benefits. Immediate exchange strategists do not consider premarital sexual relationships as merely reciprocal, but in addition expect the returns to be immediate. Where a man refuses or is unable to reward his partner, two alternatives are open to the immediate exchange strategist: partner-switching or multiple partnership. With the former the woman breaks the relationship and looks for a more lucrative friendship, as illustrated by one respondent:

> I took my first boy friend when I was 15-years-old. My present boy is the second one. At first I was small so I was not looking for anything from him. When I grew up a bit, about 17 years, I realized that I needed certain things like dresses to make myself look fine. My boyfriend was a school boy who could not give me these things so I left him and went in for someone who can give the things to me. I stayed with the first boy for about a year and a half, and with the present one for about one year three months.
>
> (19-year-old-female; middle school leaver, dressmaker)

With the second option, the woman takes on additional partner(s) who together (usually unknown to one another) meet her material needs. Although it is not a highly favoured option for most of the women, 35 per cent of respondents supported it compared with the first option which was favoured by 67 per cent. Thus, the majority were of the opinion that if the man was not living up to expectations, the best option was to leave him for someone else. The reason is not so much on moral grounds as on purely strategic ones. In a society with low levels of contraceptive use, respondents were afraid of what might become of them when they become pregnant while maintaining multiple partners. Respondents cited several instances of friends whose partners denied responsibility of their pregnancies because the men knew they had other partners.

Deferred Exchange Strategists

This group emphasizes the traditional notion of complementarity, although they accept the prevailing transactional nature of most heterosexual relationships. Unlike immediate exchange strategists they support the maintenance of currently uneconomical monogamous pre-marital relationships with a hope of change in fortune in the near future.

> I do expect material gain from sexual relationships even though I was not receiving anything from him when we started the friendship since we were all in school. You know material gain makes the relationship stronger, I must say. However, if there is a relationship devoid of material gain and there is understanding and respect for each other it is alright. This means that the woman has to work hard to help the man until he is able to get something.
>
> (21-year-old-female; middle school leaver, banana seller)

The implications of sexual exchange are quite clear. Given that many (especially young) men are not in the position to fulfil their material obligations in such friendships, and that a majority of women are reluctant to maintain relationships which are not economically viable, the risk of HIV sexual transmission is increased through multiple partnership, partner-switching, and partner-sharing.

Changing the pattern of transactional sexual culture

Although safer sex through the use of condoms is the most immediate preventive measure to reduce HIV sexual transmission, ultimately it is an overall change in sexual lifestyles that is likely to sustain HIV preventive measures. It is therefore necessary to discuss the complex issue of altering sexual lifestyles in Ghana. Changing sexual behaviour is a challenge because the behaviour is ubiquitous and highly conditioned by tradition, yet it is particularly private. In Ghana this issue is compounded by the fact that premarital sexual behaviour is influenced by pecuniary considerations, which are strongly endorsed by social norms. Unlike the promotion of condoms which derives support from the experience of family planning programmes, changing sexual behaviour is a new health educational policy. Consequently, suggesting policy recommendations is quite problematic since it involves entering a new but important field in which tried and tested intervention strategies are lacking, especially in Africa.

Economic or Normative Change?

There are at least two possible ways of influencing sexual exchange in order to bring about a substantial change in sexual lifestyles: first, given that women engage in sexual exchange mainly for financial reasons, improving their economic status to enable them to advance their occupational careers may diminish their interest in sexual networking. Second, there may be value in changing the societal norms that at present support sexual exchange with the view to encouraging young persons to engage in complimentary premarital sexual relationships consistent with the new normative pattern.

The first strategy implies the need to provide women with alternative sources of income if they are to forego the material gains derived from sexual exchange. This should be pursued by the Ghanaian government given the limited opportunities women have. However in Ghana conspicuously rich business women engage in sexual exchange for favours such as substantial bank loans, contracts, and tax evasion (Oquaye, 1980). Consequently encouraging women to reduce the numbers of sexual partners in Ghana by solely concentrating on improving the economic power of women, even though it is significantly important, is perhaps simplistic. It is suggested that interventions aimed at changing sexual lifestyles should in addition concentrate on altering the societal norms which at present strongly support sexual networking.

Social Consensus to Weaken Sexual Exchange

As pointed out by Ingham, Woodcock and Steiner, (1992), the theoretical perspectives that guide thinking behind much of sexual modification efforts in HIV publicity campaigns in western countries are basically individual-centred. For example, Bandura's self-efficacy model assumes among others 'a sense of personal power to exercise control over sexual situations' (Bandura, 1989:129). Even in the developed world where compared with Ghana or most of Africa, there is greater individual self-sufficiency and independence, there is now growing disenchantment with interventions based primarily on individuals' knowledge, beliefs and attitudes (for example, Ingham *et al.*, 1992; Romer and Hornik, 1992).

The failure of HIV prevention programmes to achieve any significant change in sexual behaviour may, in part, be attributed to the application of behavioural change models that fail to take into consideration the social context of sexual behaviour in Africa. There are certain features of Ghanaian society, as elsewhere in West Africa, which underscore the importance of community involvement in efforts at sexual behaviour change. They include the influential responsibilities and role of the extended family network, the authority of traditional rulers and other local potentates, and the existence of strong community and tribal ties.

Taken together, societal norms supporting multiple partnerism and partner switching for material reasons must be substantially weakened before individual-level change can be effected. A societal consensus perspective (Romer and Hornik, 1992) is therefore perhaps more appropriate in the Ghanaian setting. No exchange model can operate in a vacuum. Social support for a shift away from sexual exchange is crucial because individuals or partners perform within the confines of societal norms. At present a woman is considered foolish by both friends and some relatives if she maintains a materially unrewarding sexual relationship. It is not uncommon even in the rural areas as reported by Akuffo (1987), for some parents, especially mothers, to directly or indirectly encourage their daughters to engage in sexual exchange. The qualitative interviews confirmed the extent of parental support for sexual exchange ranging from overt prompting to subtle connivance. A respondent stated:

I entered into sexual relationship because when I was 16-years-old my mother refused to buy pants and other things for me. Whenever I asked her she would say: 'You're old enough; don't be asking me for such things'. So I took a partner who will be willing to provide these things.
(18-year-old-female, unemployed)

It can be seen that changing the accepted standards of sexual culture must begin by the mobilization of efforts towards a change in the existing sexual norms to be accompanied by individual change of sexual behaviour. Here, the influence of traditional rulers can be helpful.

Conclusion

For many premarital sexual relationships in Ghana, the interplay of sexual services and material needs provides a contractual relationship characterized by consumerist concerns. The specifics of the sexual relationships are regulated by unwritten but accepted cultural norms of reciprocity within a social exchange framework. In terms of HIV risk-reduction strategies, considerable emphasis needs to be placed on social and community factors which facilitate or inhibit safer sex practices. Sexual exchange is a key factor inhibiting changes in sexual behaviour in Ghana.

At the political and religious levels rhetorical emphasis is placed on fidelity without attention being given to the underlying factors which undermine it. Yet there is abundant evidence to show that material recompense for sex penetrates through the socio-sexual fabric, and underlies most pre-marital and extra-marital sexual relationships. Although the key ideas of sexual exchange are widely recognized and understood within Ghanaian society, such awareness has not been acted upon in HIV risk-reduction strategies. Policy makers need to be aware of these factors, and put sexual exchange on the public agenda.

Attempts at influencing sexual exchange can be considerably enhanced and made socially acceptable if certain traditional social norms which were contrary to consumerist relationships and can foster healthy sexual behaviour are identified and incorporated into HIV prevention strategies. They include the following: first, traditionally a man was not obliged to provide financial support for his *mpena* (girlfriend) (Sarbah, 1968). Second, as a corollary, traditional premarital relationships were characterized by complementarity and not reciprocity (Ankomah, 1992b); and third, it was traditionally the responsibility of parents to support their daughters financially until marriage.

If a critical mass of the population through integrated community-level strategies can be reached, and if societal norms can be seen to be changing with the initiative and support from traditional rulers and key opinion leaders, it is likely that sexual exchange can be substantially influenced in ways conducive to promoting safer sexual practices. Developing interventions which community members themselves understand, and in which they are directly involved, stand a high change of being effective.

References

ACQUAH, E.M. (1972) *Accra Survey: A Social Survey of the Capital of Ghana, Formerly called the Gold Coast, Undertaken for the West African Institute of Social and Economic Research. 1953–1956*, Accra: Ghana Universities Press.

AKUFFO, F.O. (1987) 'Teenage pregnancies and school drop-outs: The relevance of family life, education and vocational training to girls' employment opportunities', in OPPONG, C. (Ed.) *Sex Roles, Population and Development in West Africa*, Portsmouth: Heineman.

ANKOMAH, A. (1992a) 'The sexual behaviour of young women in Cape Coast, Ghana: The pecuniary considerations involved and implications for AIDS', unpublished PhD thesis, University of Exeter.

ANKOMAH, A. (1992b) 'Premarital sexual relationships in Ghana in the era of AIDS', *Health Policy and Planning*, 7, 2, pp. 135–43.

ANKOMAH, A. and FORD, N. (1993) *Pre-marital Sexual Behaviour and its Implications for HIV Prevention in Ghana*, Occasional Paper No. 22, Exeter: University of Exeter, Institute of Population Studies.

ASSIMENG, M. (1981) *Social Structure of Ghana*, Accra-Tema: Ghana Publishing Corporation.

BANDURA, A. (1989) 'Perceived self-efficacy in the exercise of control over AIDS infection', in MAYS, V.M., ALBEE, G.W. and SCHNEIDER, S.F. (Eds) *Primary Prevention of AIDS: Psychological Approaches*, London: Sage.

BEFU, H. (1977) 'Social Exchange', *Annual Review of Anthropology*, **6**, pp. 255–81.

BLAU, P. (1964) *Exchange and Power in Social Life*, New York: Wiley.

BLEEK, W. (1976) *Sexual Relationships and Birth Control in Ghana: A Case Study of a Rural Town*, Amsterdam: University of Amsterdam, Centre for Social Anthropology.

CHADWICK-JONES, J.K. (1976) *Social Exchange Theory: Its Structure and Influence in Social Psychology*, London: Academic Press.

CHADWICK-JONES, J.K. (1979) 'Exchange and liking', in COOK, M. and WILSON, G. (Eds) *Love and Attraction: An International Conference*, Oxford: Pergamon Press.

DINAN, C. (1983)' Sugar daddies and gold-diggers: The white collar single women in Accra', in OPPONG, (Ed.) *Female and Male in West Africa*, London: George Allen and Unwin.

EMERSON, R.M. (1976) 'Social Exchange Theory', *Annual Review of Sociology*, **2**, pp. 335–62.

HUSTON, T.L. and CATE, R.M. (1979) 'Social Exchange in intimate relationships', in COOK, M. and WILSON, G. (Eds) *Love and Attraction: An International Conference*, Oxford: Pergamon Press.

INGHAM, R., WOODCOCK, A. and STENNER, K. (1992) 'The limitations of rational decision-making models as applied to young people's sexual behaviour,' in AGGLETON, P., DAVIES, P. and HART, G. (Eds) *AIDS: Rights, Risk and Reason*, London: Falmer Press.

LITTLE, K. (1973) African Women in Towns: An Aspect of Africa's Social Revolution, Cambridge: Cambridge University Press.

MINISTRY OF HEALTH (1993) 'Reported HIV seropositive individuals as at 31 December, 1992, (unpublished), Accra: National AIDS Control Programme.

OQUAYE, M. (1980) *Politics in Ghana: 1972 1979*, Accra-Tema: Ghana Publishing Corporation.

ORUBULOYE, J.O., CALDWELL, J.C. and CALDWELL, P. (1991) 'Sexual networking in the Ekiti district of Nigeria', *Studies in Family Planning*, **22**, 2, PP. 61–73.

PELLOW, D. (1977) *Women in Accra: options for autonomy*, Algonac, Michigan: References Publications Inc.

ROMER, D and HORNIK, R (1992) 'HIV education for youth: The importance of social consensus in behaviour change', *AIDS Care*, **4**, 3, pp. 285–303.

RUBIN, Z. (1973) *Liking and Loving*, New York: Holt, Rinehart and Winston.

SARBAH, J.M. (1968) Fanti Customary Laws, London: Frank Cass.

SCANZONI, J. (1972) *Sexual Bargaining: Power Politics in the American Marriage*, Englewood Cliff, NJ: Prentice-Hall.

SCANZONI, L. and SCANZONI, J. (1976) *Men, Women and Change: A Sociology of Marriage and Family*, New York: McGraw-Hill.

STATISTICAL SERVICE (1989) *Ghana Demographic and Health Survey 1988*, Accra, Ghana Statistical Service.

Chapter 10

Positive Sex: Sexual Relationships Following an HIV-Positive Diagnosis

Gill Green

> This has been the crux of all my HIV-related problems: partners and sex
>
> (HIV-positive man, aged 24)

One would expect an HIV diagnosis to have a profound impact on sexual behaviour given that it can be transmitted sexually. Even when practising some forms of safer sex there is a slight possibility of infecting partners and, in addition, there is much public opprobrium directed at people with HIV who knowingly put other people at risk. People diagnosed with HIV thus have to re-assert their sexual identities and re-establish sexual relationships within a hostile and frightening environment related to their potential to infect others.

Concern to reduce the transmission of HIV has resulted in a plethora of empirical studies on the sexual behaviour of high-risk groups, notably men who have sex with men, male and female prostitutes, injecting drug users, and young people, as well as a large scale National Survey of Sexual Attitudes and Lifestyles of the general population (Johnson *et al.*, 1994). In comparison, the literature on the sexual behaviour of people with HIV is remarkably small, yet an understanding of this is crucial in order to inform public health policy on HIV testing, to identify the risk of transmission to HIV-negative partners and the context within which this is most likely to occur, and to provide appropriate support to people with HIV in this domain of life.

Previous studies have shown that many gay men have made substantial changes in their sexual behaviour to reduce the risk of HIV transmission (see Fitzpatrick, *et al.*, 1990), whereas only modest changes have been noted in the sexual behaviour of injecting drug users, despite marked changes in needle-sharing procedures (e.g. Bloor *et al.*, in press). There are, however, some similarities in the sexual behaviour of various sub-groups which have been studied, notably differences in sexual risk-taking with casual and regular partners. Weatherburn *et al.* (1991) reported that gay men are more likely to practice safer sex with casual than with regular partners, female sex workers usually insist on condoms during commercial sex work but not with their regular partners (McKeganey and Barnard, 1992), and heterosexual young men and women are less likely to use condoms in long-term established relationships (Wight, 1992). Women's relative lack of power in heterosexual relationships as a barrier to practising safer sex has been noted in studies of young women (Holland, *et al.*, 1991) and sex workers (Mezzone, 1993). It is still unclear, however, whether such findings are applicable to people with HIV and the extent to which their sexual behaviour is similar or different from their HIV-negative or untested counterparts.

There is substantial evidence that an HIV-seropositive diagnosis disrupts one's sex life, at least in the short term. Klimes *et al.* (1992) report that sexual relationships among people with haemophilia and their partners are adversely affected among those with HIV infection compared to seronegative controls; Catalan *et al.* (1992) note that HIV seropositive gay men experience greater sexual difficulties than HIV seronegative controls; Brown and Rundell (1990) report disruption of sexual functioning among 20 women with HIV, and McKeganey (1990) notes how some of the HIV-positive injecting drug users he interviewed had remained celibate since diagnosis. The personal testimonies of people with HIV support such findings which they relate to the fear of infecting others with HIV, the fear of being rejected by sexual partners, guilt at having unsafe sex and the loss of sexual confidence that accompanies an HIV diagnosis (O'Sullivan and Thompson, 1992; Richardson and Bolle, 1992). That some people with HIV occasionally practice unsafe sex is also consistently reported among people with haemophilia (Dublin, *et al.*, 1992), women (Hankins, *et al.*, 1993; Johnstone, *et al.*, 1990), and gay men (Weatherburn, 1993). HIV status is reported to have only a modest impact on condom use of injecting drug users and only a minority of those with HIV use them (White, *et al.*, 1993). This occurs despite a groundswell of public opprobrium which has consistently and vehemently opposed people with HIV knowingly placing others at risk. In some states of America this has been declared illegal (in Washington for example, a man with HIV was jailed for nine and a half years for having unprotected sex), and in Britain the case of a haemophiliac man from Birmingham who reportedly infected four partners affirmed that such practices would result in social ostracism. Given the moral hostility from society and the guilt and fears associated with having sex, how do people diagnosed HIV antibody positive re-establish their sexual identities?

Methods

A cohort of 66 men and women living in Scotland were asked by me (a heterosexual female) and a heterosexual male colleague about the impact an HIV-diagnosis had had upon their sex lives and sexual relationships in the short-

Table 10.1 Details of the sample

TOTAL		66
Incomplete data		7
SEX	Men	47
	Women	12
TRANSMISSION GROUP	Gay men	14
	Injecting drug users	27
	Haemophiliac	9
	Other heterosexuals	9
AGE	21–9	22
	30–9	25
	40–9	12
YEAR OF DIAGNOSIS	1983–85	15
	1986–88	26
	1989–91	18
NO. WITH AIDS		7
CURRENT RELATIONSHIPS	Has regular partner	29
	Has no regular partner	30
SEXUAL RELATIONSHIP WITH	Yes now	8
OTHER PEOPLE WITH HIV	In the past only	9
	Never	35
	Never had sex/not asked	7

and long-term. They were asked as part of a lengthy, semi-structured interview about the impact of an HIV diagnosis upon their social relationships and psychological well-being. The number included in this analysis is 59, as three respondents refused to talk coherently about their sexual behaviour and four were not asked.[1] The cohort was recruited from hospital clinics, voluntary agencies, self-help groups and prisons. It included both men and women (mostly men) and people from all transmission groups. The largest group were injecting drug users, but also included were gay men, people with haemophilia and people probably infected heterosexually (see Table 10.1). The age range was 21–49, the majority in their late twenties or early thirties. All the respondents were white. The interviews were conducted in 1991/92, and some respondents were therefore interviewed only a few months after diagnosis and others almost eight years after. The majority of the cohort were asymptomatic, but some were ill, and seven had an AIDS diagnosis. The diversity of the sample was apparent in their sexual identities, sexual orientation, sexual experience and current sexual situation. There was a vast range in experience ranging from five who were sexually inexperienced at diagnosis (two of whom remained so at time of interview) to several of the women who had in the past worked as sex-workers and some of the gay men who reported having had hundreds of sexual partners. This was often reflected in their willingness to talk about sex, some clearly feeling uneasy on this topic, whereas others were relaxed and fluent. In addition, their current situation varied dramatically with half the sample having a resident or non-resident partner, some who had been in the relationship for over a decade, and half having no partner, including many who had never had one. About one-third reported that they had had a relationship with a partner who was also HIV seropositive (nine in the past and eight currently). In about half of these relationships they had met their partner when both had already been diagnosed HIV-positive.

Getting accurate information about sex is never easy, particularly from people who carry the sexual stigma of an HIV diagnosis. It is a highly sensitive area particularly for those respondents who had restricted access to sex through being in prison or had lost the desire for sex through being too ill. We also realized that the information collected would be largely affected by both the respondents' and the interviewers' gender and sexual orientation. So a simple checklist was used, and none of the items were mandatory. This included number of casual and regular partners pre- and post-diagnosis, safer sex practices pre- and post-diagnosis, context in which safer sex was not practised, how they informed partners of their HIV status, HIV status of partners, emotional impact of HIV on relationships, periods of celibacy, reproductive history, overall impact of HIV on sex lives and sexual relationships, and the impact this had on life. Given the diversity of the sample, respondents were encouraged initially to use their own definition of safer sex, and were then asked what they meant by this.

Some limited data were also collected on the sexual behaviour of a group of HIV-negative controls who were matched pair-wise with the HIV-positive cohort by age, gender and transmission group. This data included the number of regular and casual partners pre- and post-testing, whether any behaviour change had resulted from having an HIV test, and whether they currently practised safer sex with regular and casual partners.

Table 10.2 Sex life following diagnosis

Celibate since diagnosis	
Too fearful of infecting others	6
Celibate or impotent for limited period(s)	
Immediate response to diagnosis; failure to achieve safer sex (e.g. burst condoms); following break-up of relationship; in response to an AIDS diagnosis; ill health.	19
Sex life deteriorated in quantity/quality	
Self or partner concerned about infection; dislike safer sex; ill health; guilt.	13
Little disruption	
Denial by self (and sometimes partner too); confident in practice and efficacy of safer sex.	14
Missing data	7

Findings

Table 10.2 shows the ways in which an HIV diagnosis may affect sexual behaviour. The majority of the sample (38 out of 52) reported that their sex life had been disrupted to a greater or lesser extent and had been either celibate or had no libido for at least a limited period, or found sex less fulfilling than prior to diagnosis. A small number reported that they had been celibate since diagnosis. In the main, those who selected this path were older than average, had no partner at diagnosis, did not view sex as an important part of their identity or had previously experienced difficulties with sexual relationships. As one person with haemophilia said, 'I just want a drink and a fish supper. Females don't interest me.' Their desire for sex was less than their fear of transmitting HIV to a partner; according to a male heterosexual respondent, 'I just couldn't do it. She wanted me to but I didn't. You can't risk passing it on to somebody else' (Male heterosexual). Many reported that they had had no sex for a limited period either as a result of loss of libido or deciding to become celibate. For most in this category this was the time immediately following diagnosis and lasted from two months to three years.

> After my diagnosis I had no sex for one year. I just had no libido whatsoever.
>
> (Gay man)

> At first I was like men were a no-go area. I feel bitter towards them and I'm really quite rude to them now. I'm not nice to them. They get the message and go away.
>
> (Female heterosexual)

A few people who initially responded to diagnosis by having no sex, reported in the interview that they had subsequently overcome their initial fear of sex, and three people who had since met HIV-positive partners reported that they were enjoying better sex than ever as it was more intense and caring. Others became temporarily celibate in response to specific events such as a condom bursting or a relationship ending and for some, such events were the precursor to total celibacy. 'A few times condoms have burst and I could see he was terrified so I stopped. We're more like friends now' (Female injecting drug user). Some at more advanced stages of HIV disease find they lose their libido in response to an AIDS diagnosis or the onset of prolonged ill-health. 'Going out in Glasgow used to be sexually motivated but I can't go and chat up someone and say I have AIDS' (Gay man).

Another group continued to have sex following diagnosis but reported it was less frequent with both regular and casual partners and/or less fulfilling. This group mostly had partners when diagnosed and either they or their partners were fearful of sex, as the following quotations illustrate:

We did have a good sex life. We were sort of doing it all the time. We used to make love but after the diagnosis it changed. I did not want to be touched. I didn't enjoy it. I would just lie there and think hurry up. I was just worried about infecting him.

(Female injecting drug user)

The sexual side of things are really iffy. He said he is not scared but I think he is. He is like scared to really kiss me.

(Female injecting drug user)

Several people reported disliking safer sex; one female sex worker said that using condoms made her feel as if her partner was a punter, others lived in fear of a condom bursting and, with the exception of some of the gay men, most respondents felt that non-penetrative sex was not 'full sex' and therefore unsatisfactory. A few others alluded to the guilt they felt associated with the public opprobrium about people with HIV enjoying any sort of sex life. 'I know a lot of moral society would be against me sleeping with anyone so I have that guilt' (Person with Haemophilia).

Only one-quarter of the sample reported little disruption to their sex lives following diagnosis, and consisted of two quite distinct groups. The majority were those who denied or were not aware of the implications of an HIV-positive diagnosis and failed to modify their sexual behaviour, and sometimes failed to inform their partner. The others who reported little disruption often had no regular partner at diagnosis and were either already practising safer sex and continued to do so, or found the transition to safer sex following diagnosis relatively unproblematic. Their confidence in the efficacy of safer sex, and their ability to enjoy it, enabled them to continue their sex life with minimum disruption. With time, a few of the respondents who initially responded to diagnosis by becoming celibate or losing their libido became confident practitioners of safer sex and learned to enjoy sex again.

There were few differences between men and women with regard to sex life following diagnosis, but there were some marked differences between transmission groups. Both male and female injecting drug users reported much less disruption to their sex lives than other groups (11/22 injecting drug users compared to 3/27 in other groups).

The impact of diagnosis upon sex life clearly has implications for safer sex practices and the risk of transmission. Those who become celibate have no risk of transmitting the virus sexually to others, whereas those who deny the implications of diagnosis and fail to modify their behaviour are at risk of transmitting the virus to sexual partners. Respondents were asked whether they always practised safer sex with regular and casual partners.[2] In regular relationships less than one-half (18/44) said that they consistently practised safer sex, whereas in casual relationships more than one-half (15/25) said they did.

Table 10.3   Context in which safer sex did not occur with regular and occasional partners

REGULAR PARTNERS	OCCASIONAL PARTNERS
No evidence of wishing to infect partner	No evidence of wishing to infect partner
In nearly all cases partner is aware of HIV status	In most cases partner is not aware
In some cases partner also HIV-positive	Does not know HIV status of partner
Denial	Denial
Lack of information	Lack of information
Practical problems with safer sex	Practical problems with safer sex
In most cases with partner's consent	No emotional attachment
Partner wants commitment	
Desire to have child	
Love	

Within regular partnerships the women in the sample were observed to be less likely to practice safer sex than the men due to their relative lack of power in sexual relationships. An extreme example of this is one woman who reported being raped. There were also some marked differences by transmission group. Injecting drug users were much less likely than other groups to practice safer sex, reflecting the tendency of some to deny their potential to infect others sexually. Gay men were the most likely to say they consistently practised it, perhaps reflecting the greater ability of members of the gay community to communicate about sex, and their greater readiness to modify behaviour in response to HIV.

The difference between sex with regular and casual partners is well illustrated by comparing the context in which safer sex was not always practised (see Table 10.3). We found no evidence for a favourite tabloid myth of people with HIV willingly infecting others to 'get their revenge' on society with either regular or casual partners. On the contrary, most people reported changing their sexual behaviour in response to diagnosis and generally claimed to practice safer sex most of the time with both regular and casual partners. They were very much more likely to practice safer sex with both regular and casual partners than the HIV-negative control group that were interviewed.

In most cases the HIV status of self and partner was known in regular partnerships, although there were a few instances where this was not the case; regular partners were not always told immediately after diagnosis, and new regular partners were often not told until the relationship was firmly established as, 'I was not willing to expose to him that I was positive or negative because I was not quite sure how the relationship was going to work out' (Female heterosexual). Many respondents in new relationships also delayed disclosure fearing that they would be rejected by their new partner (although the number of actual rejections reported were few). In general, the HIV status of self and partner was not discussed in occasional or transitory relationships, although it was sometimes known if both mixed in the same social circles. In both regular and casual relationships where both partners were known or thought to be HIV-positive, safer sex was less likely to occur.

Another reason for not always practising safer sex in regular and occasional relationships was related to the denial of HIV status. People diagnosed with HIV sometimes took a while to modify their sexual behaviour and adopt safer sex. In regular relationships, denial was often practised by both parties who were sometimes prepared to acknowledge the diagnosis in everyday life but ignored the implications in their sex life. With casual partners temporary denial was occasionally the cause of one-off unsafe sex encounters often when away from home, or when drunk.

Another factor hindering the practice of safer sex, at least for some of those diagnosed in the mid-1980s, was lack of information about routes of transmission of HIV. One man was just told 'not to bander it about' and only when he overheard a conversation in the treatment clinic did he realize he could pass it on to his partner. Others did not realize how serious an HIV diagnosis was, and thought it more akin to hepatitis B, and some were not told that unsafe sex with an already HIV–positive partner could result in cross-infection.[3]

A further obstacle to the practice of safer sex with both regular and occasional partners related to practical difficulties particularly in the use of condoms. The majority of respondents claimed not to like them and a minority said they or their partner could or would not use them. Women often found it impossible to negotiate sustained condom use particularly within long-term relationships. 'I would rather we used condoms all the time but sometimes he comes in drunk and before you know it we are just having sex' (Female injecting drug user).

The most important contextual factor affecting sexual behaviour with regular and occasional partners relates to trust and commitment. In regular partnerships unsafe sex generally takes place in a loving and caring relationship with the full knowledge and consent of both participants, whereas with occasional partners, sex most usually occurs outside a committed and trusting relationship. With regular partners, HIV generally becomes a part of that relationship and decisions about the relationship sometimes are given higher priority than the risk of HIV transmission. In moments of high passion and excitement, the closeness some derived from unsafe sex was more important than the possible consequences. About one-half of those with HIV concordant partners, for example, thought that lack of restrictions on their sexual behaviour was worth the risk of cross-infection. In discordant couples, it was reported by some that their partner encouraged them to have penetrative sex without a condom in order to make them feel more committed to the relationship. Others mentioned that their partner wanted to have a child or that their partner considered HIV to be a joint problem, and if the person they loved was infected they may as well be too. In some cases where the couple was discordant, the decision to have unsafe sex was reported to be against the wishes of the HIV–positive partner who reported feeling guilty afterwards.

Patterns and implications

Three sexual 'careers' following diagnosis may be identified among this cohort of people with HIV in Scotland. The first is the path of celibacy, the second that of denial of the possibility of infecting others and failure to modify behaviour, and the third is the path of behaviour modification which enables a sex life to continue while placing HIV-negative partners at minimal risk. Amongst the small group of individuals studied here, injecting drug users were more likely than other groups to choose the path of denial which may be related to their having different thresholds and assessments of risk. Most people with HIV eventually choose some compromise between celibacy and denial and take the path of safer sex. Some, but not all, who follow this path are able to enjoy a fulfilling sex life, but many feel guilty or become ill and opt for celibacy. Those that are more sexually confident seem to be most likely to negotiate this third path successfully, including gay men whose sexual culture empowers them to practice safer sex. The path an individual chooses may vary with time following diagnosis. Many initially opt for celibacy or denial but may later feel sufficiently sexually confident to adopt the third path. And those who initially respond by practising safer sex may change in response to changing circumstances, such as a new partner or onset of illness or specific events like a burst condom.

There is evidence to substantiate previous research findings that an HIV diagnosis disrupts sexual behaviour as most respondents reported having less sex and enjoying it less than prior to their diagnosis; this was mostly related to their fear of infecting their partner. There is little evidence to support claims that a majority of people with HIV practice unsafe sex. The great majority claimed to practice safer sex with both occasional and regular partners most of the time, and comparison with a control group of people who tested HIV-seronegative suggests that most people modify their sexual behaviour following an HIV seropositive diagnosis. A substantial minority, however, claimed to have practised unsafe sex on at least one occasion, and it was reported that this mostly occurred with partners' knowledge and consent. In this respect, the context in which unsafe sex occurs is different with regular and occasional partners, and places regular partners at slightly greater risk. Earlier findings that injecting drug users are more resistant to change in their sexual behaviour than other groups, particularly gay men, are confirmed; an HIV-seropositive diagnosis seems to have had a much less disruptive effect on the sex lives of injecting drug users in the sample than other respondents. These findings from a Scottish-based sample thus broadly confirm some results from other studies conducted in other parts of Britain and in the United States.

A number of public health implications derive from these data. First, HIV-testing may reduce the amount of unsafe sex by people with HIV, as those that know their positive status have less sex, and safer sex than those who test HIV-seronegative. The data also suggest that knowledge of HIV status does not prevent some people with HIV having unsafe sex some of the time, and identifies groups which could perhaps be targeted for behavioural change. Since unsafe sex often occurs with the full knowledge and consent of partners, intervention in this area is more likely to be effective if the focus is upon the couple rather than the HIV-positive individual. Couples should be given more information about the risks of transmission, assistance in planning when to have children, and sex counselling to increase their ability to practice and enjoy safer sex. The current censorious moral climate about the sex lives of people with HIV infection is, however, unlikely to encourage people with HIV from seeking such advice.

Notes

1 The four respondents that were not asked included two who had lived in institutions since diagnosis and had restricted access to sexual relationships, one whose wife had been infected by the respondent and died of AIDS a few months prior to interview, and one who had fallen asleep before the questions about sexual behaviour.
2 It is quite rare to report those who *always* practice safer sex. Most surveys report those who 'usually' or 'sometimes' do. We used 'always' in order to probe for 'even one' occasion when safer sex was not practised. Therefore the figures for those not always practising safer sex include several respondents who reported only one instance of 'unsafe sex'.
3 Unsafe sex between two people who are both HIV seropositive may result in re-infection. The significance of this is, however, much debated amongst clinicians.

Acknowledgements

Thanks are due to the respondents who were prepared to discuss intimate, and highly stigmatizing, areas of their lives, to Steve Platt who conducted almost half of the interviews, and to Steve Green, Miriam Guthrie, Helen Mien and Anne Pinkman for their assistance with respondent recruitment.

References

BLOOR, M. FRISCHER, M., TAYLOR, A., COVELL, R., GOLDBERG, D., GREEN, S., MCKEGANEY, N. and PLATT, S. (in press), 'Tideline and turn? possible reasons for the continuing low HIV prevalence among Glasgow's injecting drug users', *Sociological Review*.

BROWN, G.R. and RUNDELL, J.R. (1990) 'Prospective study of psychiatric morbidity in HIV seropositive women without AIDS', *General Hospital Psychiatry*, **12**, pp. 30–35.

CATALAN, J., KLIMES, I, DAY, A., GARROD, A., BOND, A. and GALLWEY, J. (1992) 'The psychosocial impact of HIV infection in gay men: A controlled investigation and factors associated with psychiatric morbidity', *British Journal of Psychiatry*, **161**, pp. 774–8.

DUBLIN, S. ROSENBERG, P.S. and GOEDERT, J.J. (1992) 'Patterns and predictors of high-risk sexual behavior in female partners of HIV-infected men with hemophilia', *AIDS*, **6**, pp. 475–82.

FITZPATRICK, R., MCLEAN, J., BOULTON, M., HART, G. and DAWSON, J. (1990) 'Variations in sexual behaviour in gay men', in AGGLETON, P. DAVIES, P. and HART, G. (Eds) *AIDS: Individual, Cultural and Policy Dimensions*, Basingstoke: Falmer Press.

HANKINS, C., GENDRON, S., LAMPING, D., LAPOINTE, N., KIELO, J. and GAUTHIER, S. (1993) 'Does an HIV-positive test result improve a woman's sex life?' Poster (PO-D20–3974) presented at IXth International Conference on AIDS, in Berlin.

HOLLAND, J., RAMAZANOGLU, C., SCOTT, S., SHARPE, S. and THOMSON, R. (1991) 'Between embarrassment and trust: Young women and the diversity of condom use', in AGGLETON, P. DAVIES, P. and HART, G. (Eds) *AIDS: Responses, Interventions and Care*, London: Falmer Press.

JOHNSON, A.M., WADSWORTH, J., WELLINGS, K. and FIELD, J. (1994) *Sexual Attitudes and Lifestyles*, London: Blackwell.

JOHNSTONE, F., MACCALLUM, L. and RIDDELL, R. (1990) 'Contraceptive use in HIV-infected women', *British Journal of Family Planning*, **16**, pp. 106–8.

KLIMES, I., CATALAN, J., GARROD, A., DAY, A., BOND, A. and RIZZA, C., (1992) 'Partners of men with HIV infection and haemophilia: Controlled investigation of factors associated with psychological morbidity', *AIDS Care*, **4**, 2, pp. 149–56.

MCKEGANEY, N. (1990) 'Being positive: Drug injectors' experiences of HIV infection', *British Journal of Addiction*, **85**, pp. 1113–24.

MCKEGANEY, N. and BARNARD, M. (1992) 'Selling sex: Female street prostitution and HIV risk behaviour in Glasgow', *AIDS Care*, **4**, 4, pp. 395–407.

MEZZONE, E.J. (1993) 'An exploration of the difficulties encountered by female sex workers in negotiating safer sex with non-commercial partners: A qualitative approach', paper presented at the 7th Conference on Social Aspects of AIDS, London, University of the South Bank.

O'SULLIVAN, S. and THOMSON, K. (Eds) (1992) *Positively Women: Living with AIDS*, London: Sheba Feminist Press.

RICHARDSON, A. and BOLLE, D. (Eds) (1992) *Wise Before their Time: People with AIDS and HIV Talk about their Lives*, London: Harper Collins.

WEATHERBURN, P., HUNT, A.J., DAVIES, P.M., COXON, A.P.M. and MCMANUS, T.J. (1991) 'Condom use in a large cohort of homosexually active men in England and Wales', *AIDS Care*, **3**, 1, pp. 31–41.

WEATHERBURN, P., DAVIES, P.M., HICKSON, F.C.I., COXON, A.P.M. and MCMANUS, T.J. (1993) 'Sexual behaviour among HIV-antibody positive gay men', poster (PO-D20–3996) presented at the IXth International Conference on AIDS, in Berlin.

WHITE D., PHILLIPS, K., MULLEADY, G. and CUPITT, C. (1993) 'Sexual issues and condom use among injecting drug users', *AIDS Care*, **5**, 4, pp. 381–91.

WIGHT, D. (1992) 'Impediments to safer heterosexual sex: A review of research with young people', *AIDS Care*, **4**, 1, pp. 11–23.

Chapter 11

A Telling Tale: AIDS Workers and Confidentiality

Rosaline S. Barbour

Due to the stigma attached to HIV/AIDS — and to particular groups of people who have been disproportionately affected (such as gay men and injecting drug users) — the issue of confidentiality has been paramount in AIDS work. This is evidenced by the attention given to the topic in counselling textbooks (see Bor, Miller and Goldman, 1992; Dilley, Pies and Helquist, 1989). As Zonana (1989: 226) states:

> Confidentiality remains an integral and time-honoured feature of the therapist-client relationship. The emergence of HIV has brought many new challenges to this issue, and as long as HIV-infected individuals are stigmatised, discriminated against and refused treatment, the confidentiality of such data (i.e. relating to serostatus) will remain a dilemma.

Although, to a certain extent, confidentiality and its limits are defined by statute in Britain for some professional groups, the situation varies from one country to another.[1] For some professional groups 'the only guidelines may be ethical principles promulgated by the specific professional organisation' (Zonana, 1989:220).

Even where restrictions, regulations or guidelines exist, they cannot hope to cover all eventualities or permutations involved in the complex web of relationships and circumstances surrounding work with HIV seropositive individuals, in in-patient and out-patient treatment settings, the family and in the community. Similarly, such guidelines cannot cover all staff working or associated with the complex organizations in which 'confidentiality' is located, which ensures that its realisation, if ever possible, is problematic.

The notion of confidentiality is socially constructed: thus there are both inter- and intra-professional variations with regard to its interpretation and implementation. There are also important variations with regard to institutional responses, as well as amongst individual workers and clients. There has been a tendency for enormous value to be placed on confidentiality, while very little attention has been given to studying the context within which workers respond to issues surrounding the making and breaking of confidences. This chapter constitutes an attempt to move away from a taken-for-granted notion of what confidentiality involves, and to examine some of the wider ramifications of 'confidence work' for staff.

The data described here was collected in the course of a project funded by the Medical Research Council. In-depth interviews were carried out with 153 workers and volunteers providing services for people with HIV or AIDS in a range of statutory and voluntary health and social care agencies. Workers were interviewed about their experiences of AIDS-related work in both specialist AIDS Units or AIDS community teams, as well as integrated units (e.g. a haemophilia unit, a maternity unit, an infectious diseases ward and drugs projects). Just over half of the sample were involved in providing hands-on nursing care in the hospital, hospice or in the community — either as care assistants, auxiliaries or nurses of various grades. The remainder were ancillary staff (such as domestics and receptionists) or other professional staff, including doctors, social workers, physiotherapists, dieticians, occupational therapists, drugs workers, chaplains and clinical psychologists. Interviews took place during 1991 and 1992 in four Scottish cities — Glasgow, Edinburgh, Dundee and Aberdeen — selected to reflect different patterns of epidemic spread and service response.

The 'telling tale' of the chapter's title relates to the imparting, maintaining and breaking of confidences within the context of HIV/AIDS work. As will be shown, perceptions of confidence boundaries are constantly open to revision and re-negotiation in problematic situations or at points of tension.

Organizational structure and policies

In the course of the study it became clear that requirements about confidentiality varied considerably depending on whether staff worked in specialist AIDS Units, integrated wards or generic teams. Certain wards become known very quickly in local parlance as 'the AIDS ward' and staff could give examples of patients who were very reluctant to come to the in-patient unit, since this would automatically identify them to outsiders and potential visitors as having AIDS. Staff highlighted such features as the wording on wall plaques at the entrance to Units as being important in fostering or dispelling these associations.[2]

Even when they are hospitalized and terminally ill, patients may not have shared their diagnosis with all members of their family and staff often described how they walked a tightrope, trying to establish and keep in mind who knew and who did not know, and guarding against letting slip any details which might arouse relatives' suspicions. Surprisingly, perhaps, some patients on designated AIDS wards, or even residents in the AIDS Hospice, managed to keep their diagnosis secret from some visitors — a testimony to staff skills with regard to confidence work.

Where people with AIDS are nursed alongside other patients in an integrated infectious diseases ward or on a general ward, there is the added possibility that other patients will find out and disclose the identity of seropositive patients through ward gossip, or forment concern about transmission. In the course of the research, I was told many horror stories, most of which related to early hospital-based responses to the care of people with AIDS. Most of these stories portrayed staff members as over-reacting by dressing up 'in spacesuits', leaving yellow polythene bags outside rooms, hanging up notices on doors saying 'Isolated', supplying separate cutlery or crockery and making provision for separate toilet arrangements. Such horror stories clearly have a dual function for staff. They demonstrate how far services have progressed since these early days of the epidemic and the hysteria which sometimes characterized agencies' responses, but they also underline the ever-present potential for disclosure inherent in the taking of special precautions or in the implementation of administrative policies.[3]

Where universal precautions were routinely adhered to this presented few problems. However, staff in some general care settings admitted that they sometimes forgot to don aprons or gloves at the start of ward rounds, and to do so when caring for people with AIDS, they considered, could alert the person in the next bed to the fact that this patient was different in some way. In specialist units, all members of staff (including ancillary staff, such as porters and domestics) were aware that all patients or clients were HIV-seropositive. Since all of these specialist units had been set up from scratch, an ability to handle confidentiality had been seen as an important criterion in the selection of staff. Although interview questions may be poor predictors of actual behaviour once in post, the selection interviews did allow managers as prospective employers to stress the importance of confidentiality as a working principle. In generic teams or integrated wards, however, interesting variations emerged in the policies regarding the information passed to staff. Where distinctions were made in relation to access to information about patients' HIV serostatus, these generally reflected professional boundaries and existing organizational hierarchies. Thus, on some general wards, only the qualified staff would be party to this information. On other wards, however, nursing auxiliaries would also have access to this information by virtue of their inclusion in ward meetings. Thus, policies governing the disclosure of information relating to patients' serostatus reflected the patterns already in operation with respect to sharing information. Ancillary staff in the same settings, however, did not have access to information about clients' serostatus.

Some interesting questions were raised by the implementation in some settings of a policy involving confidentiality between team members of equal status. In this situation only an individual's key worker or key workers would be notified of his/her HIV serostatus. Drugs projects, in particular, favoured this approach, but this was also the approach used in the maternity unit included in the study. In practice, it sometimes proved difficult to maintain confidentiality:

> If a member of staff gets a needle-stick injury from one of our patients who is seropositive it is my experience that the patient would want the information to be given to the health care worker. They wouldn't mind provided they didn't go and tell everyone else. But the problem is, it's going to be very hard to keep confidentiality because if everyone knows that Nurse Bloggs pricked her finger off that [patient] and then the next day she is sitting there with red eyes because she's been crying all night because she thinks she's going to die . . . everyone knows then that the [patient] is infected.
>
> (Interview with Doctor — Integrated Maternity Unit)

Policies about the maintenance of confidentiality could also have implications for team relations and support:

> We have a policy here whereby we don't actually tell other team members if people are . . . what their HIV status is — so that then becomes difficult because then I have to explain some reason why I've still got this person who's not a very regular attender at the project — why I've still got this person on my caseload . . .You can't always get the support you need with a case because of the confidentiality thing: sometimes that's a barrier.
>
> (Interview with Drugs Worker)

Lay and professional notions of confidentiality

Confidentiality can extend to cover not only a client's HIV serostatus, but can encompass information about drug use, social and emotional problems, family dynamics and sexual identity. Moreover, maintaining confidentiality with regard to his or her serostatus may be a secondary concern for the client. There may even be a disjuncture between lay and professional disclosure norms. Clients may not be used to hiding very much about their lives and may live in areas where many residents already know someone who is seropositive or who takes drugs. Stigma can be relative, and is certainly context-dependent.

 This is not to argue, of course, that staff should routinely disclose such details, as reactions will vary enormously between individuals. However, this is to underline the importance of variations between individuals' expectations about confidentiality. Several staff members recounted their irritation with patients who had happily disclosed their seropositive status to hospital porters, for example, 'after all the trouble we had gone to to keep it confidential'.

The imparting of confidences by clients may be a source of considerable professional pride for workers, who value their ability to get clients to open up and give them an opportunity to exercise their counselling skills. Clients may recognize and exploit this 'professional vanity' with a resulting exacerbation of professional and interpersonal rivalries. In one setting, workers recounted how they had reluctantly come to the realization that certain clients had told the same story 'in confidence' to several members of the team.

Whereas workers often expressed concerns that clients might be discriminated against if other individuals or services were made aware of their HIV serostatus, clients might seek to use a seropositive test result to attempt to obtain more or better services: to secure positive discrimination. Whereas HIV/AIDS workers may wish to restrict access to this information, clients may wish to let as many workers as possible know, in the hope that they can thereby maximize their access to allowances and any other preferential treatment reserved for known seropositive individuals.

There was also some tension between workers who interpreted their role as being to secure everything possible for clients in the way of allowances and those who took a wider perspective, citing the existence of resource limits and pondering the implications for the client body as a whole of zealously pursuing benefits for particular clients, regardless of notions of relative need. In addition, professionals are not solely responsible for the clients on their caseloads, but also have a wider remit. It has been argued that HIV/AIDS workers have a responsibility to provide support to those affected directly *and* indirectly by the virus (Coxon and Carballo, 1989). This raises two main issues for workers: firstly their general public health responsibilities and, secondly, their responsibilities towards particular individuals who may be at risk. HIV/AIDS workers may be aware, for example, that a particular client is continuing to drive a car while suffering from dementia or some other condition potentially involving erratic behaviour. They may become party to details about a forthcoming drugs shipment or information about drug dealing or possession of weapons.

A related concern was the discomfiture of some workers when regaled with details such as 'how many fingers a client had chopped off of how many people', accounts of housebreaking expeditions, stories about shop-lifting. Many confidences come unbidden, but some are more welcome than others. The provision of extraneous and disturbing detail is, of course, unlikely to be a feature specific to HIV/AIDS work. Nor do such revelations necessarily involve large numbers of clients on any one worker's caseload — although they did tend to be related to drug users, who formed the single largest client group for workers in the Edinburgh and Dundee study locations.

Reactions to these revelations evidence a significant culture gap between workers and clients. Many of the workers interviewed expressed a desire to minimize barriers between themselves and their clients and to be able to empathize with clients as people rather than cases. Such dramatic disclosures forced them to acknowledge the existence of this gap, and, consequently, the limits with regard to the ability to cut down barriers and to fully empathize with clients. References to such unwelcome confidences were accorded prominence in workers' descriptions precisely because they were so vivid and because they raised so many questions for staff — for example, is the information 100 per cent accurate in any case? Workers find such confidences burdensome and were taking the opportunity of partially unloading or sharing them within the relative safety of a research interview with its own code of confidentiality.

One popular staff strategy for dealing with unbidden confidences relied on anticipating the imparting of such confidences and heading them off. 'After a while you get to know when certain conversations are leading round to descriptions of criminal activity and you say you do not want to know about it' (Interview with Doctor — Specialist AIDS Unit) This strategy, however, depended on familiarity with the work and client group and was, therefore, not an approach which could automatically be used by new members of staff.

Problematic issues

Patients continuing to take unprescribed drugs — or 'extras' — while hospitalized was a topical issue in all in-patient settings. This was of considerable concern to staff since, as well as having legal implications, taking extras could have repercussions for the clinical management of patients and, ultimately, a nurse's registration could be at stake. Appealing to team as opposed to individual responsibility was a popular approach — however, it does rely on clients being in a fit state to process this information, to understand the distinction being made and realize the implications of what the worker is saying:

> But one of the things that I'll do, if I go into somebody's room and they'll say, 'You can't tell anybody — it's between me and you'. I'll say, 'I have to tell somebody' — I just have to say, 'No, we're a team in here and I can't guarantee. I have to take it back to the team if it's something that I think is relevant to your care . . .' I caught one of [the patients] taking extra tablets one day but she was in a really bad state at the time and I was frightened in case she OD'd and I had to say to somebody, but I felt so creepy and, you know, a clype.[4]
>
> (Interview with Nurse on AIDS ward)

Ancillary staff in specialist units — the only units where they were party to sensitive information about clients' HIV-serostatus — put a similar emphasis on confidentiality as a value. However, such members of staff experienced particular problems in relation to handling confidentiality. Because of their close day-to-day contact with patients, staff such as domestic workers were frequently singled out by patients wishing to impart confidences. Ancillary staff tended to be older than qualified staff and it was suggested by some respondents that this might be a factor which made them more attractive to patients as persons in whom to confide:

> We're closer (than in previous jobs) to patients too. They tell us — they tell me — a lot and I think they see me as a kind of mother figure (laughs) . . . granny, and they tell you a lot of things they wouldn't tell other people — not even the nursing staff they'd tell.
>
> (Interview with Domestic in a designated AIDS Unit)

This was not something which had occurred in previous jobs, where ancillary workers' role had been confined largely to cleaning. As a result, dealing with the demands of confidence work was a new experience for these members of staff. Moreover, because of their association with relatively menial tasks, patients might see domestic workers as less of a threat: 'You get people that they come and they tell you a lot of their problems, know, they talk to us, I think, quite a lot — sort of open up to us. I feel, ken,[5] I mean, I think because we're just the ladies that go about with the hoover and the dust . . .' (Interview with Domestic in a designated AIDS Unit). Ancillary staff were also more likely than were the professional staff to live in the same public housing schemes as clients, or to know them socially through friendship networks. Thus the potential for breaches of confidentiality was greater. Whereas professional staff might have attended training courses with an experiential element, and would certainly in the course of their training have encountered hypothetical situations in which there were dilemmas about confidentiality, domestic workers were more likely to have to formulate a response to a new problem *in situ*. The following extract illustrates how guidelines were established in response to a difficult situation:

> One of the other domestics got into that kind of situation and she was really worried sick about it, you know. It had to do with someone dealing drugs . . . She couldnae pass it on because it was told to her in confidence, and 'What would the person think' if she did. But she did. We talked it out with her . . . and after that they (the nursing staff) said to us, 'If you're told anything or (if) they say, "Now I don't want you to tell anybody else", you must say, "Well we work as a team, so, therefore, we would have to go and report it."'
>
> (Interview with Domestic worker in a designated AIDS Unit)

Invoking team responsibility mirrored the strategy used by qualified staff in dealing with similar issues. Notwithstanding guidelines from nursing staff and the permission contained therein to disclose information passed to them in confidence, ancillary staff continued to have difficulty in deciding when such an approach was appropriate:

> A young lad that was in here, he says to me, 'Would you look in on me later?' I says 'Why?' He says, 'When I take that medicine sometimes I have a fit and they're quite violent.' Well, he was going to have a shower and everything and I didn't keep that to myself. I went and saw the person in charge and they had a nurse come . . . He hadn't told them. They didn't know that the medication could work that way. And I apologized to him and he says, 'No, it's alright', he says, 'I just didn't think to tell anyone else', and I apologized that I did. I wouldn't normally break confidence, but for things like that you must do, because he could have fell on the stone floor when he's having his shower, so, and that kind of thing, you know.
>
> (Interview with Domestic worker in a designated AIDS Unit)

When it came to workers' responsibilities towards other individuals, there was considerable disagreement amongst staff as to how this should be handled. A particularly difficult issue for staff to resolve concerned the responsibilities of the HIV-seropositive individual to current or previous sexual partners.[6]

The issue of how to deal with refusal to disclose seropositivity to sexual partners relates partly to individual workers' personal moral codes or ethical standpoints. However, the range of responses to broadly similar scenarios suggested that differences in workers' professional backgrounds and work settings could lead to somewhat different approaches being adopted.

A nurse in a designated AIDS ward provided the following description of workers' responses:

> I remember the most difficult time was a patient who was married with a family, who was HIV-positive and still having a sexual relationship with his wife but refused to tell his wife his HIV status. And confidentiality was extended to everybody and therefore we weren't allowed to divulge it, and I remember having a lot of problems dealing with it myself, because my gut reaction was, 'No — it was unfair.' But you're tied by the ethics of the job and obviously you've got to be guided by them . . . There was a lot of us feeling the same way at the time and I think we all just kind of slowly worked through our feelings about it. Some people agreed with him totally that it was his business and therefore if he didn't want to tell anybody he shouldn't. Other people had the feeling, 'No, — that was extremely irresponsible and extremely unfair . . .'
>
> (Interview with Nurse working in a designated AIDS Ward)

Although this situation gave rise to vigorous debate about the rights of the individual, staff responses were confined to discussion about the issues involved.

A community psychiatric nurse working on a drugs project, by contrast, had taken a more active role:

> I've got a client who's seropositive and, well, his girlfriend must suspect . . . he's being seen here so often. She just doesn't want to think about it. I've tried to set up sessions with her to talk about it and give her the opportunity to talk about any concerns she has about Davy's drug use. And you'd think that'd eventually drop the hint — let her come to a gradual realization. She must know, but she won't admit it even to herself . . . But some of the other (staff) in the team say, '*He's* your client — that's not your problem', so I don't know . . .'
> (Interview with community psychiatric nurse — Drugs Project)

This worker was attempting to create a situation where she could work towards admission of risk and, potentially, subsequent realization and disclosure.It may be that staff who work in the community are more likely to view their responsibility as extending to all members of the house-hold. Staff members who define their remit thus, may also see it as part of their role to tackle and attempt to resolve situations involving couples in 'a con-spiracy of denial' (Lippmann, James and Frierson, 1993). Another worker reported:

> There's a woman at the moment. Her ex-husband is HIV positive and she's just burying her head in the sand. I mean, I've tried — I've written to her and I've gone round to her flat but she was out . . .
> (Interview with Health Advisor — GUM Clinic)

Significantly, this worker was employed in a Genito-urinary Medicine (GUM) Clinic, a setting which has a history of involvement in contact tracing for other sexually transmitted diseases.

As well as being party to information that partners do not have, staff may be party to information that professionals outside of their immediate team do not have. As in their work with relatives, workers have to sort out exactly who is party to which pieces of information. An HIV/AIDS diagnosis and the resultant confidence work can thereby impact on the normal reciprocities involved in collegial working relations. AIDS workers, for example, expressed annoyance over requests for information from other agencies or other departments in the same hospital. These were usually requests such as those from social work departments asking for results of urine tests (which would determine drug use) or questions about clients' HIV serostatus from paediatricians or labour ward midwives elsewhere in the same hospital. Workers reported that they had always refused to provide this information, citing as justification either profes-sional boundaries or the importance of universal precautions. Although caus-ing irritation, such requests were not problematic for workers in terms of formulating responses — they viewed such requests as inappropriate and dealt with them accordingly.

Confidence work takes place within the often fraught atmosphere of inter-professional rivalries and can exacerbate any tensions or conflicts involved. Writing about work with the terminally ill, Vachon (1987) commented that dealing with confidentiality was often dependent on notions of superior communication skills and rivalry. Just as sharing one's own confidences with another is an expression of trust, so too can be the sharing of confidences second-hand. Where outside workers are members of the same professional group as AIDS workers requirements for restraint may be particularly burdensome. Although support was generally forthcoming from other members of multi-disciplinary teams, professional staff did not always have a colleague to hand from the same discipline, and sometimes only someone of similar professional background could provide the particular mixture of support and information which was required. Workers, like clients, may be identified through their placement in specialist units, and the implications of indirectly revealing a client's serostatus to a colleague working elsewhere may compromise workers' ability to elicit support. If, in seeking support, a specialist HIV/AIDS worker circumvents such potential problems by withholding information which would normally be passed to a colleague providing support, she or he may be seen as implying that the colleague cannot adhere to the professional group's own code of conduct, which may be viewed by non-specialist workers as encompassing confidentiality concerning HIV serostatus. Thus, appeals for support to colleagues outside the AIDS field may serve merely to confirm these other workers' suspicions that AIDS workers regard themselves as an elite with superior skills in confidence work.

Confidence work as situated activity

Confidentiality is, by its very nature, largely invisible. It is thus hard to demonstrate that it is being properly observed. Interviews conducted as part of this study afforded workers an opportunity to identify instances which they saw as their successes. In each of three practice settings in separate cities, workers cited the case of a couple, both HIV-seropositive and both attending as outpatients, neither of whom was aware of the other's serostatus. While lamenting the poignancy of such a lost opportunity, workers in each case underscored their satisfaction regarding the observance of confidentiality, by adding words to the effect of, 'that's good confidentiality by anyone's standards'.

The imparting of confidences does not take place within a vacuum. Certain situations foster the conditions favourable to making disclosures — for example, night duty, administering lengthy treatments or simply day-to-day contact. Confidence-sharing episodes are characterized by intimacy and are often highly-charged exchanges. Staff members often commented that they were sharing more of themselves with people with AIDS than they had done with other people with whom they had worked in the past. This might take the form, as one nurse put it, 'of sharing the ongoing trivia of one's day-to-day life' or it could be more extensive, and staff may or may not set limits around what they discuss with patients. It is not surprising that some become emotionally — and even, on occasion — romantically involved.

Although certain circumstances may facilitate confidence sharing, they are not a prerequisite, and the imparting of confidences seems to remain an essentially spontaneous affair. Clients will confide when they feel the need — when they are upset, for example. Thus their choice of who they disclose to may be apparently indiscriminate — it may simply be a case of whoever is around at the moment when a client feels the compulsion to open up. Ancillary staff may therefore be just as likely to receive confidences as professional staff, by virtue of their protracted and regular contact with patients. Although the ancillary staff who had found themselves in this position attached the same value as did professional staff to confidentiality as an ideal, they were more likely to have to rely on informal support when coping with what they had been told, and were less likely to have had access to counselling courses.

Conclusions

Certainly blanket policies regarding confidentiality are unhelpful. To extol confidentiality as an unassailable and all-encompassing principle has precisely the value of an advertising slogan — absolute virtues make poor guidelines for action. Meanwhile, workers continue to wrestle with the complex, varied, and unpredictable demands which confidence work makes of them. At the very least, wider acknowledgement of the far from straightforward nature of confidentiality and confidence work may stimulate more open discussion and lay the groundwork for developing the professional support which is so crucial for those working in the field of HIV and AIDS.

Notes

1 See Pollak, 1992, for national variations with regard to notification procedures and disclosure practices).
2 It must be emphasized that, once breached, confidentiality cannot be retrieved, and the potential for unintentional disclosure is ever-present. For example, staff in specialist units have to be constantly vigilant when answering the telephone as merely confirming that an individual is a patient in a designated AIDS Unit can signal to others that they are HIV-seropositive.

3 Turnbull, Dolan and Stimson (1993), in their account of the separate care and treatment of HIV-seropositive prisoners, report that they are subject to both 'physical and emotional privations'. Although this is an extreme case, it nevertheless highlights the dramatic — and perhaps unintended — consequences of organizational arrangements which involve segregation or other restrictions.

4 'Clype' is a Scottish word. It is a pejorative terms and refers to somebody who tells tales, or who is a gossip. What is significant about this comment is that it demonstrates the strong belief in confidentiality as an ideal — even in the face of such complicating factors.

5 Scottish for 'you know'.

6 Anticipating problems of this nature, Swedish regulations stipulate that seropositive individuals must sign a contract stating that they will inform all sexual partners of their HIV status (Mansson, 1990). Given that ultimate control over such sensitive information rests with the client — who is the only person in possession of all the details — it is difficult to see how this could be enforced in practice and how practitioners could distinguish between compliant and non-compliant clients.

References

BOR, R., MILLER, R. and GOLDMAN, G. (1992) *Theory and Practice of HIV Counselling: A Systemic Approach*, London: Cassell.

COXON, A.P.M. and CARBALLO, M. (1989) 'Research on AIDS: Behavioural perspectives', *AIDS*, 3, pp. 191–7.

DILLEY, J.W., PIES, C. and HELQUIST, M. (1989) (Eds) *Face to Face: A Guide to AIDS Counselling*, AIDS Health Project, San Francisco: University of California.

LIPPMANN, S.B., JAMES; W.A. and FRIERSON, R.L. (1993) 'AIDS and the family: Implications for counselling', *AIDS Care*, 5, 1, pp. 71–8.

MANSSON, S.A. (1990) 'Psycho-social aspects of HIV testing: The Swedish case', *AIDS Care*, 2, 1, pp. 5–16.

POLLAK, M. (1992) 'Organising the Fight against AIDS', in POLLAK, M., PAICHELER, G. and PIERRET, J. (Eds) *AIDS: A Problem for Sociological Research*, London: Sage.

TURNBULL, P.J., DOLAN, K.A. and STIMSON, G.V. (1993) 'HIV testing, and the care and treatment of HIV-positive people in English prisons', *AIDS Care*, 5, 2, pp. 199–206.

VACHON, M.L.S. (1987) 'Team stress in palliative/hospice care', *The Hospice Journal*, 3, 2/3, pp. 75–103.

ZONANA, H.V. (1989) 'The duty to protect: Confidentiality and HIV', in DILLEY, J.W., PIES, C. and HELQUIST, M. (Eds) *Face to Face: A Guide to AIDS Counselling*, AIDS Health Project, San Francisco: University of California.

Chapter 12

AIDS Policies in Kenya: A Critical Perspective on Prevention

Charles Nzioka

The Kenyan response to the AIDS problem has been somewhat conservative and clearly lacking foresight. Other than the formation of AIDS control committees at various levels, screening of donated blood in hospitals, unco-ordinated activities by various organisations and the establishment of an AIDS programme secretariat within the Ministry of Health, not very much has been done for a problem of this magnitude. It should be noted that the various AIDS control committees in this country are mainly composed of medical personnel which is very unfortunate.

(Dr. Omondi Oyoo, *The Daily Nation*, 9 January, 1992:16)

In the recent past, numerous discourses have represented Africa as a continent engulfed in an AIDS inferno, with a population on the verge of extinction. In this continent, where the dominant means of HIV transmission is unprotected heterosexual sex (Mann, 1988a; 1988b), the World Health Organization (WHO) estimates that by 1994, 10 million Africans will have acquired HIV infection, compared to an estimated 2 million in the whole of the industrialized west. By the year 2000, up to 750 000 cases of AIDS may be occurring on the continent annually. Such figures leave little room for optimism, and far from being helpful to people in Africa, only foster a sense of hopelessness.

Similar projections made in western countries like Britain with the advent of HIV/AIDS in the early 1980s have, however, not been matched by subsequent incidence. At present, questions are being raised as to whether such estimates were products of moral panic, given the potentially devastating impact of AIDS. Indeed, the controversy now is whether the enormous resources that were committed to HIV/AIDS awareness and prevention then were justified, and whether these resources could not have been more fruitfully utilized in providing health care facilities for other curable diseases. It would, however, appear that both the proponents and critics of this mass anti-HIV/AIDS campaign have justifiable cases. Proponents argue that the now observed shortfall between the early high projections, and the observed cases up to the present, represents the success of this investment. From this perspective, this investment was not in vain because potential infections and possible deaths due to HIV/AIDS have been averted. Critics, however, argue that such an investment was in the first place unnecessary, given that it was based on wrong statistics and moral panic, and that these resources could have been better utilized. For them, the massive investment in the HIV/AIDS control campaign was misdirected.

The relatively *ad hoc* nature of AIDS control programmes in most African countries inhibits any clear assessment of the actual investment that has gone into them, as well as their impact. The AIDS control terrain is characterized by many players, ranging from central to local governments, through foreign and local non-governmental organisations to individuals. It is a landscape characterized by conflicts of interest, competition, and non-accountability. If there have been any major achievements in managing the epidemic, their impact is obscure. The mass media continues to portray Africa as a continent engrossed in a fathomless HIV/AIDS quagmire, where the prospects of a decline in the rates of HIV/AIDS are bleak. Anti-AIDS efforts in Africa are therefore waged against a background of despair and pessimism and a chronic shortage of resources.

Africa clearly has her share of HIV/AIDS, and it is certainly not the intention to deny this. With infection rates of 12 to 13 per cent being reported in some villages, such as in the Kagera region of Tanzania, and in the Rakai district of Uganda (Wawer, *et al.*, 1991), HIV/AIDS seems well established in some parts of the continent. However, reports of people who had been 'diagnosed' as HIV seropositive being *cured* as soon as their material conditions were improved raises questions. In a continent where disease prevalence is high, preventive medicine is still a preserve of few (Kalibala and Kaleeb, 1989), and where food shortages, hunger and starvation are endemic, vulnerability to disease is a necessary consequence. The high prevalence of HIV/AIDS in Africa needs therefore to be examined, at least in part, from a political economy of poverty and deprivation both at the micro- and macro-level. At the national level, the reluctance or inability of many African governments to marshall enough resources of their own to tackle HIV/AIDS has forced them to leave open the doors to international philanthropic forces eager to assist in controlling AIDS. This has created a fertile ground for HIV/AIDS to be socially and politically constructed in a variety of ways. If it is the case that the extent of HIV/AIDS in Africa is misrepresented, and that the frightening statistics on the continent are a fabrication, it is also the case that this is part of the price to be paid for charity. It is against this background that this chapter is written.

HIV/AIDS in Kenya

The first case of AIDS in a Kenyan who had not travelled out of the country was reported in 1984. Since then, reported cases of HIV/AIDS have continued to swell, rising from 843 in 1985 to 5949 by March 1989 (Ministry of Health, 1989). By the close of 1992, there were well over 33 902 reported AIDS cases (Kibwana, 1992) and at present, an estimated 750 000 Kenyans are said to be HIV positive but asymptomatic. While the main mode of HIV transmission in Kenya appears to be unprotected heterosexual sex, there may also be homosexual transmission, but information is lacking. Most of those affected fall between 20 and 40 years of age, and the rate of infection in both sexes is about equal. Urban areas are the most affected. Mombasa leads in the number of HIV/AIDS cases, followed by Nairobi and Kisumu. The situation in the rural areas where over 85 per cent of the population live is not quite clear, although there are fears that the strong urban-rural kinship linkages offer paths of transmission. In a projected national population of 30 million people in 1996, the number of adult HIV infections is estimated at 1.7 million (Ministry of Health, 1992b: 3). These estimates, if true, illustrate the scale of the HIV/AIDS problem in Kenya, which the government will need to address in the not too distant future. With a cure or vaccine being a dim prospect, the only feasible AIDS control measures seem to lie in behavioural change.

With those mostly affected being the young and economically productive people, HIV/AIDS is not simply a medical problem, but a social and economic one. People with AIDS and HIV may also require long-term intensive care, occupying a sizeable number of available hospital bed spaces, and creating a demand for palliatives. This is certainly an extra expense which the Kenya government, whose health care budget is already overstrained, can hardly afford. Put together, these factors underscore the importance of swift implementation of policies and programmes that can check the rapid spread of AIDS.

As elsewhere, responses to HIV and AIDS in Kenya have taken place in three main fields: first in health education and preventive medicine; second in development of an infrastructure to provide treatment and care for people with AIDS and HIV; and third, at the cultural level where dominant meanings about AIDS are established (Watney, 1991:5). These areas have, however, become sites of intense socio-political friction. It is in this context that recent anti-AIDS campaigns in Kenya will be examined.

Initial Responses to HIV/AIDS

Once the problem of AIDS was identified as a legitimate concern, the Kenya government decided to establish a national infrastructure under which all matters and activities pertaining to AIDS control could be organized and co-ordinated. The first step was the establishment in 1985 of the National AIDS Committee (NAC) in the Ministry of Health, whose mandate was to make an appraisal of the situation in the country and advise the government on how best it could be tackled. It was not, however, until 1987 that the committee started its work (see Ministry of Health, 1992b). Soon after that a diagnostic surveillance and reporting infrastructure was established which entailed screening all blood donated in the country. Before then, blood was only screened for hepatitis and syphilis. A five-year Medium Term Plan (MTP) for AIDS control, was also formulated, and in this plan the government decided to invite the World Health Organization (WHO) to assist in the mobilization of resources in the fight against HIV/AIDS. This culminated in the launching of the Kenya National AIDS Control Programme in 1987 whose major components included health education, epidemiology, clinical services, laboratory and blood transfusion services. To promote public health education campaigns, and to create awareness of the disease and its prevention, the AIDS Programme Secretariat (APS) was established. Since then, success has been reported in certain areas, though in others, the progress and achievements have been rather less noteworthy. According to the then Minister for Health, Mwai Kibaki, as of November 1991, among the most salient achievements of the national exercise of controlling AIDS in Kenya was a near 100 per cent screening of donated blood in the national, provincial, district and mission hospitals. Second, there had been an establishment of counselling and nursing procedures, as well as guidelines for protection of health workers. Third, weekly broadcasts in 18 local languages were being aired regularly on all the radio stations and there were some programmes on the national government-owned television station. Fourth, awareness-enhancement seminars had been held right across the country to sensitize administrators and opinion leaders to the problem of AIDS and finally, there were attempts to decentralize the AIDS Programme Secretariat with a view to making its services more accessible nationwide (see Kibaki, 1991).

This success has, however, not been made without problems. Notable among them has been shortages in qualified personnel, as well as a lack of HIV-antibody testing kits and other equipment. However, the major bottleneck to the planning, and implementation of AIDS control programmes in Kenya, and possibly many other African countries, has been a lack of funds. With Kenya having an overstrained health budget, and with the problem of HIV/AIDS coming as an additional burden, there has been a tendency to over-rely on externally donated funds to finance the AIDS control programme (Kibaki, 1991). However, with the deep economic recession gripping much of the western donor countries, the amount of foreign assistance coming into the country has been dwindling. This diminished funding has severely compromised much of the local HIV/AIDS project planning and implementation. Programmes have had to be abandoned altogether or be managed with severely reduced budgets. In addition, western aid has, in recent years, assumed unprecedented political dimensions. As a political tool, such aid has been used to arm-twist African governments and subdue them into adopting or conforming to western democratic ideals and beliefs. The amount of aid given has largely been proportional to the level of adherence and conformity to these beliefs. For countries that have been slow in changing their political systems to conform to western political prescriptions, the resulting cuts in aid have resulted in severe economic hardships. Kenya has not been spared in the process, and this is exemplified by the limited finances at the disposal of her AIDS control programme.

Foreign donations have also had the undesirable effect of suppressing local fund raising and management initiatives. Instead of the government exploring the possibilities of raising funds locally either from individuals, companies, churches, and community organizations, it has continued to depend almost entirely on foreign donor agencies. Modest as such contributions might be, they would help ease the present over-reliance on external donor funds, and reduce the funding uncertainties that have characterised programmes in the past. This could also represent an initial step towards developing a national capacity for the self-financing of anti-HIV/AIDS campaigns. As Omondi Oyoo warns:

> For a problem threatening to wipe us out, we cannot rely entirely on foreign funding as is the case now. It is very critical for Kenyans to indigenously support the projects.
>
> (Oyoo, 1992a:7)

Critics of the national AIDS efforts, however, point out that the National AIDS Committee's dismal performance cannot be attributed solely to lack of funds. They argue that, there is need for the Committee to review and set its priorities, as much of the resources at its disposal have been in the past on activities tangential to, rather than central to, AIDS control. As one critic put it:

> It is sad to say so, but the committee has been largely a failure. The more-than Shs 800 million the committee had at its disposal has already been spent on hotel bills, air fares, purchase of vehicles, generous personal allowances and fuelling and servicing project vehicles, which most of the time do not do anything related to AIDS control.
>
> (Oyoo, 1992b:7)

Regardless of the merits of these allegations, it is enough to say that the government must look into ways and means of raising funds locally for the AIDS control campaigns, while also ensuring that there are sufficient checks and balances on the National AIDS Committee to ensure its financial accountability.

Charles Nzioka

Health Education and Condom Use Promotion

In the first five year AIDS control plan (1987–91), the Kenya Ministry of Health observes *inter alia* that:

> Through information and education, people will be helped to make informed decisions in adopting life styles that do not favour transmission and spread of AIDS.
>
> (Ministry of Health, 1988:16)

The health education and information strategy which is the pillar of the anti-AIDS campaign in Kenya is based on a framework of rational choice. The inherent assumption is that individuals can and will make rational decisions which take full account of the 'perceived severity of the condition, the level of risk, the costs and benefits of alternative behaviour changes and the presence of cues to action' (Ingham, Woodcock and Stenner, 1992: 163). A distinction, however, needs to be drawn between information dissemination and health education. Information supply involves making available facts about HIV/AIDS, while health education is a more elaborate and integrated approach and may involve informed exchange between the information supplier and consumer (Moerkerk and Aggleton, 1990).

The Kenya government, it would appear, has decided to concern itself with information supply especially after its sole mouth-piece the Kenya Broadcasting Corporation (KBC) became an autonomous body in 1992 as part of the new policy of privatizing public corporations. In theory, if not in practice, all advertisements carried on the KBC's radio and television are supposed to be paid for, so as to enable the corporation to generate revenue for self sustenance. Prior to 1992, the government could freely use KBC's broadcasting facilities to promote its activities including HIV/AIDS awareness programmes. The Ministry of Health, however, now seems to place anti-HIV/AIDS 'advertisements' on the KBC radio and television network, rather than programmes. These advertisements aired or televised are singular in their lack of detail. However, HIV/AIDS programmes placed by private companies and Non-Governmental Organizations (NGOs) on the same network are more elaborate, detailed, informative and analytical. Whether this is related to the cost of air time on these networks, or to the design of the advertisements is difficult to tell. The government through the Ministry of Health will need to get involved in health education rather than in placing advertisements and distributing posters if its campaign will have a significant impact.

Levels of HIV/AIDS awareness are reported to have increased dramatically from very low levels in 1985, to well over 90 per cent in 1992 (Muturi and Nzyuko, 1988; Ministry of Health, 1992a). These impressive statistics, however, reveal little if anything about changes in sexual behaviour and the adoption of safer sex practices. Such statistics also provide little insight into people's views on the quality and quantity of such anti-AIDS information. Before becoming overly complacent about these initial, seemingly high levels of HIV/AIDS awareness, much more should be established about what people actually know, about HIV/AIDS, how they get to know it, and what sense they make of such information. After all, over the same period that HIV/AIDS awareness is reported to have been rising, the number of HIV/AIDS cases has also been on the increase.

A variety of reasons have been advanced for this increase. For example, Muturi and Nzyuko (1988) argue that knowledge of the risks involved in certain lifestyles may not provide sufficient deterrent effects unless individuals are confronted with concrete evidence of the dangers involved, for instance having a friend with AIDS (see also Jackson, 1988). They see knowledge of, or interaction with, people with AIDS/HIV as a deterrent to unprotected sex. Second, it has been claimed that the message-content of many AIDS education campaigns has been camouflaged in incomprehensible language, lacking sensitivity to culture, lay beliefs, traditional values, and emotional needs. Third, the mass media have been accused of sensational reporting, which places emphasis on death and frightening statistics, something designed more to sell newspapers than to increase public knowledge and understanding of HIV/AIDS (Panos Dossier, 1990). In consequence,

> faded posters now the subject of graffiti and sometimes reversed and used for other propaganda such as football matches, hang apologetically from their stands. AIDS leaflets, read and unread, understood and misunderstood, lie idly in any number of public venues and valid questions remain in the minds of many.
>
> (Laver, 1988: 282)

Having information about the risks involved in a certain activity may be a necessary condition for behaviour change, but information *per se* is certainly not sufficient to bring about lasting behavioural change, and particularly change in sexual behaviour. The uniqueness of each person's life, his or her social-economic standing, and his or her gender, are but a few of the variables affecting individual sexual behaviour. It is certainly the case that

> Individuals do not simply absorb information and respond logically by modifying their health-related behaviour. Rather, people actively 'make sense' of new ideas they encounter by assessing them in the light of pre-existing beliefs, interpreting them accordingly, and fitting them with what they already know.
>
> (Wilton and Aggleton, 1991: 149)

The present view by the Ministry of Health and the National AIDS Committee in Kenya, that a standardised advertisement or poster will mean the same thing to all people, and that it will facilitate certain sexual behavioural changes is simplistic in the extreme. For safer sex messages to be effective, they must engage with,

> . . . not only lay beliefs about the origins, aetiology and effects of the syndrome, but also socially, culturally, ethnically, religiously and politically specific significations of sexual desire and practice
>
> (Wilton and Aggleton, 1991: 150)

The core message in most AIDS education campaigns is safer sex practices. However, within government circles, safer sex is viewed as synonymous with condom use. This behaviour modification approach (Moerkerk and Aggleton, 1990) built on the rational choice framework, assumes that people will use condoms if they know the risks of unprotected sex, and if the condoms are available, either at modest prices or free. To ensure that condoms are available commercially, and at affordable prices, all imported condoms have been exempted from customs and excise duty. However, a packet of *Durex* in Nairobi containing three condoms costs anything between Kshs. 27 and Kshs. 30,[1] — a price still considered high by local standards. Second, to ensure that free condoms are available, the government has tried to procure free supplies of condoms from donor agencies. These condoms are then distributed freely in family planning clinics throughout the country. However, these clinics, especially in the rural areas, are few and far between, making them physically inaccessible to a large segment of the population. Additionally, condoms are distributed by hospital staff, and the fact that condoms may be associated with promiscuity may inhibit many from asking for them. Moreover, the time spent in the long queues in these public health institutions may discourage many from going for them if that was their only need. Third, the quality of the condoms given out freely is not guaranteed. These condoms are reported to rupture easily, something authorities attribute to poor handling and storage facilities in the generally hot environment. From my interviews with people with AIDS and HIV and other consumers, fears were expressed that these free condoms could even be the possible sources of HIV, which is part of an orchestrated move to reduce local populations. Some condom consignments received as donations also arrive long after the 'use by date'. Finally, by using only the family planning clinics as distribution points for condoms, the government unwittingly discriminates against the wider population. The reason why condoms are channelled through family planning clinics also relates to the moral sensitivities that surround public promotion of condom use. The prospect of generating open hostility from some religious bodies, like the Catholic church, or upsetting parents has inhibited the government from espousing condom use as a formal government policy (Ministry of Health, 1992a). To promote condoms as a family planning prophylactic is thus an attempt to circumvent this moral obstacle. However, according to government figures, the demand for condoms has quadrupled since 1985 from about 5 million a year to over 20 million in 1992 (Ministry of Health, 1992). Whether this recorded rise in demand for condoms was a response to the fear of AIDS is difficult to discern. If, however, this was an adequate index of sexual behaviour change, we could safely conclude that Kenyans have adopted safer sex *en masse*. These raw statistics, are, however, difficult to interpret as condom sales do not equate with condom use.

While making condoms available has remained a priority area of government, the dynamics of condom use have been viewed as a private domain of the individual(s). The ultimate decision to use or not to use condoms is regarded as a territory for the couples, and therefore not within the ambit of government intervention programmes. The assumption that prudence will override emotions (Dawson, 1991) has however been challenged (Silverman, 1990). Condoms are not used simply because they are available. The negotiation of condom use in any relationship is a complex process calling into play a variety of psycho-social and economic issues. Studies in the west reveal that condom use, especially in heterosexual relations, can be problematic, and perhaps even more so than in male homosexual relations. It is noted that, in heterosexual relations, 'men and women lack a context in which to engage in issues of sexual practice in ways which are distinct from moral notions of "good" and "bad"' (Wilton and Aggleton, 1991:152).

If heterosexual sex is viewed as natural, normal, spontaneous and unpremeditated, in which erotic feelings, emotions and passion override any ethical considerations, the act of getting out a condom in the heat of the moment may seriously impair a relationship (see also Holland *et al.*, 1991). First, the condom implies premeditation of sex. Second, it disrupts the rhythm of the act, and finally, it raises moral questions of trust and the character of the sexual partner. Moreover, in heterosexual relations, there is a complex interplay of social power-relations which dictate whether or not condoms can be used (Wilton and Aggleton, 1991). These lifestyle modification approaches (Moerkerk and Aggleton, 1990; Watney, 1991) demand an understanding of the psycho-social and economic factors that come into play in the sex negotiation process.

HIV/AIDS Counselling

HIV/AIDS counselling is an integral part of the whole disease management process. Counselling enables people with AIDS and HIV, and their friends or relatives, to adjust to the demands of the condition. However, HIV counselling is an area that has not, until recently, received much attention in Kenya. By 1992, national guidelines for counselling services had been developed, though in some areas of the country, 'some participating groups were still in the process of collecting data for use in improving some aspects of the curriculum' (Ministry of Health, 1992b:81). The number of personnel trained in counselling, let alone HIV counselling, is remarkably low in Kenyan medical institutions. The government does not have a training programme for counsellors, so it relies heavily on training offered by NGOs for its health professionals. NGOs such as the African Medical Research Foundation (AMREF), the Red Cross Society and churches take the lead in training government health officials. By 1992 nationwide, some 500 health professionals had received a two week HIV counselling course, and counselling had also been integrated into the clinical management seminars for nurses, doctors and clinical officers (Ministry of Health, 1992b). The national organization of this service had, however, been somewhat *ad hoc*. By failing to train many counsellors, the burden of having to counsel those with HIV/AIDS increasingly falls on doctors and nurses. The consequences of this are two-fold: first, scarce medical skills are used on an activity that would otherwise have been done by a non-medical specialist; second, the quality of counselling given by the medical speci...list may not be guaranteed given that this is not his or her speciality. As a rational way of using government resources, and in particular, the limited medical personnel in public health care institutions, counselling services should be strengthened as part of the overall HIV/AIDS management exercise. The present neglect of HIV/AIDS counselling is, perhaps, a consequence of the National AIDS control infra-structure being dominated by medical professionals. From my field observa-tions, some of these medical professionals do not immediately see and appreciate the value or the rationale of having trained counsellors work alongside them in HIV/AIDS management. By nurturing a narrow view that HIV/AIDS is a medical problem with a medical solution, they regard others without medical skills as trespassing into their jealously guarded territory. Such a mistaken notion needs to be radically altered in the best interests of the people with AIDS and HIV. The government will need to put more resources into the provision of HIV-counselling training, and play a more salient role in providing this essential service.

Identification of Risky Groups

Women who sell sex are largely victims of economic deprivation and as such by-products of the local capitalist economy (Nelson, 1987). Yet, these women not only embarrass the political elites, they comprise one group that the political elite would evidently prefer to forget (Watney, 1991). To the political elite, prostitution is not seen and explained from a political-economic framework, rather, explanations are sought in theories grounded in the sociology of deviance. Consequently, prostitution is explained and justified through reference to personal weakness and class inadequacy (Cohen, 1991). In the personality framework, prostitution is seen as a personal attribute, a naturally-occurring, stable deviant behaviour, immutably fixed and not culturally determined (Watney, 1991). In the class framework, which is rarely acknowledged in public, prostitution is seen as deriving from belonging to a certain social class whose behaviour is socially deviant. It is also the case that Kenyan society is largely patriarchal, and dominant sexual beliefs which have informed HIV and AIDS education campaigns are based on male chauvinistic ideals. These ideologies of male dominance represent female prostitutes as the reservoir of sexually transmitted diseases and HIV/AIDS. With the advent of HIV/AIDS in Kenya, politicians, researchers and government officials targeted female prostitutes as the problem, making eloquent speeches on how these prostitutes should be avoided if 'people' (as though prostitutes were not people) were to protect themselves against HIV/AIDS.

Medical researchers were then mandated to initiate surveillance and epidemiological studies, which were not so much intended to investigate the existence of seropositivity in the prostitute population, as to confirm the HIV infection rates. Working on the *a priori* assumption that the prostitutes were already infected, their task was simply to find out the numbers infected. This saw many of these HIV/AIDS studies concentrated on 'low class' prostitutes living in the slum areas of major towns such as Nairobi, Mombasa and Kisumu. Although no justification was ever advanced for the choice of these particular sites and samples, two reasons emerge: one, that most researchers are indeed part of the elite class, and the squalid living conditions in the slums provided easy comparisons with their affluent lifestyles, easily reinforcing the class framework theory. Second, the choice of the sample provides a basis for expressing power relations between the elite researcher and the sample. Because prostitutes are not the intended consumers of these research findings, because their class positions deny them the educational, political and economic power to do so, such findings cannot easily be invalidated, as there can be no challenge to them.

This situation compares with the one in the west in which for a long time, AIDS and HIV was regarded as a disease of male homosexuals, injecting drug users and immigrants. Through concerted efforts, the gay community was able to challenge and reverse this unfounded, negative and distorted public views. Political agitation for gay rights would not, however, have succeeded had it not been for the intellectual and economic resources at its disposal. In Kenya, however, those regarded as belonging to the risky categories are largely the victims of deprivation. These people, who include truck drivers, bar-attendants, vegetable vendors and hawkers, lack the affluence and influence necessary to counter biased mainstream views. Their struggle to survive leaves them with no surplus time and resources to launch counter-reactionary campaigns, making them easy targets of attack and discrimination. Being marginal groups, they become favourite samples for elitist researchers who seek only to confirm their biased theories and hypotheses — findings which precede the actual research. Such findings, which reinforce the graphic images of people down-trodden by

HIV/AIDS , and in real need of help, provide additional evidence in support of the government, research institutions and charitable organizations bid to raise funds locally and abroad. The political elites themselves, however, are not subject to the same degree of medical surveillance.

AIDS and the political elite

Increasingly, the line between politics and AIDS in Kenya seems to be fading. The requirement that all HIV/AIDS related research in Kenya be sanctioned by the National AIDS Secretariat (which is basically manned by political appointees), and by the Office of the President, where such sanction can be denied if, in the opinion of this office, the research might jeopardize public interest, demonstrates how politicized HIV/AIDS is in Kenya. Effectively, this amounts to the removal of research from the control of academics and professional researchers, where research quality is assessed on the basis of theoretical adequacy, methodological rigour, and ethical standards, and its placement within the 'lay' domain, where political considerations now play the decisive role. What may be regarded as 'good' research thereby becomes synonymous with what goes down well with local elite thinking, and with what promotes the *status quo*.

The elitist stance towards risk taken by politicians in Kenya is reflected in a new culture of invulnerability that seems to dominate the political representation of HIV/AIDS. One politician after another has died of AIDS; however, the politicians' concerted efforts have been directed more to denial than acknowledgement. In effect, the Kenyan politicians' culture of invulnerability defines and approves what is conceived of as the common good for Kenyans. The political elite has demonstrated yet again, how historical assumptions and references to HIV/AIDS as a disease of certain socially constructed categories of people has informed their attitudes to the management of the epidemic. By refusing to be drawn into the anti-AIDS campaign, political leaders in Kenya have re-affirmed the symbolic interpretation of the disease as belonging to the lower orders in a class conscious society. With the advent of AIDS a decade ago, the same politicians were reluctant to publicly acknowledge the full scale of the epidemic on the pretext that such publicity could cause irreparable damage to such vital sectors of the economy such as tourism. Little acknowledgement was, however, made of private fortunes in such ventures, allowing personal interests to be tactfully couched in nationalistic phrases.

This served to legitimate the Kenyan politicians' trait of arrogance and hostility towards HIV/AIDS. In Uganda, a neighbouring state to Kenya, which for over a decade has been locked in a protracted civil war, and has a fragile economy dominated by foreign investments, aid and trade, the political leadership has been much more responsive to the HIV/AIDS problem. For example, Uganda's National AIDS Control Programme falls under the Office of the President, and the President is personally actively involved in these campaigns. However, in Kenya the daunting task of organizing AIDS control programmes has been relegated to less powerful civil servants in the Ministry of Health and to a host of NGOs. However, problems of co-ordination, duplication, and competition between them abound.

The puritan approach adopted by Kenya's political leadership stems in part from the national political culture in which political leadership still revolves around personality cults. By refusing to be drawn into public discourse on HIV/AIDS and sexuality which are arguably immoral, these political leaders strive to present images of infallibility. Moreover, Kenyans are familiar with the catch-phrase 'leave politics to politicians' now slowly being added to the national political vocabulary, which can imply that HIV/AIDS is the concern for medical professionals as much as matters of sexuality and morality are the legitimate concerns of religious leaders. By adopting such a position, politicians are able to justify to Kenyans their aloofness from the HIV and AIDS discourse. At the heart of this political ambivalence lies some latent clergy/politicians rivalry. Rarely acknowledged is the fact that, in a country like Kenya, religious organizations and leaders wield enormous political influence. So strong is this influence, that in the event of conflict of opinion between political leaders and church leaders, it is the politician who turns out to be the loser. For the Kenyan politician, the stakes of indulging in HIV/AIDS discourse might be too high to mitigate involvement. HIV/AIDS discourse invariably raises questions of morality, which happen to lie within the theological or religious domain. Faced with the prospect of a clash with the clergy in an area outside their jurisdiction, and on which they (politicians) know very little, the possibility of losing the popularity they so dearly cherish, and with threats of possible revelations of their hidden sexual lives, the rewards of silence appear much more attractive.

Given the limited gains to be made from publicly participating in the HIV/AIDS discourse or campaigns, politicians have chosen to either avoid them or get involved only when it is part of their official duties to do so. For example, a recent seminar organized for Kenyan parliamentarians attracted only 23 participants from a pool of 200 legislators. Even more disheartening was the fact that participants comprised only 2 cabinet ministers, 4 assistant ministers, while the other 16 were back-benchers (see Njenga and Muita, 1991). Sadly, even the Minister for Health could not find time to attend such a meeting. Moreover, despite President Moi's populist politics, it would appear that AIDS is one of those items on his political menu which he has found quite unpalatable. In the seven years since AIDS became an acknowledged problem in Kenya, apart from a few isolated instances, the President only found time to mention AIDS in public on 12 December 1991.[2] Saying that AIDS will kill *all of us*, President Moi observed that:

AIDS was a reality and the myth by some people that the disease did not exist should be discarded. He urged Wananchi (citizens) not to believe in any trial drugs as there was no known cure for AIDS at present. The only cure was one's moral values; to abstain. The President said many lives would be lost as the AIDS scourge takes toll.

(*The Standard*, 13 December 1991:2)

In a letter published in *The Daily Nation* (Nyairo, 1992:7), a concerned Kenyan argues that it is time that HIV-seropositive prominent Kenyans and politicians 'came out' as a way of changing the present culture of invulnerability. Noting that in Uganda, Phil Lutaya, a Ugandan Musician of international fame, had returned from his sojourn in Belgium to Uganda and made it known he had AIDS, something which other personalities like the American actor Rock Hudson did in 1985, and other US sports personalities like Magic Johnson and Arthur Ashe did still later, it is disappointing that no prominent Kenyan had disclosed seropositivity. Even the former President of Zambia, Kenneth Kaunda, had the audacity to declare publicly that his own son had died of AIDS, but the situation among politicians in Kenya has been one of pretending in public all is well.

The popular view among government critics has been that AIDS threatens the cord of national life, and just as the security of the state is controlled through the highest office on the land, so should be AIDS. This view is so strong that even members of the Kenya National AIDS Committee subscribe to it, a clear testimony that all is not well with the present arrangement. An independent review mission evaluating the performance of the National AIDS control programme in 1992 observed that a National AIDS Council should be established and 'housed in the Office of the President with a secretariat and members being Permanent Secretaries from other relevant ministries, donors, NGOs, major private companies and prominent individuals' (Ministry of Health, 1992b). This view is echoed by Dr. Omondi Oyoo who observes: 'The control and prevention of AIDS threat should be co-ordinated from the Office of the President to mobilise all sectors of the society' (Oyoo, 1992a:16). From public comments in the local newspapers, there seems to be a common view among critics that the present National AIDS Committee has outlived its purpose, and should be disbanded because its poor record can no longer justify its existence.

The AIDS phobia in this culture of elite invulnerability is so considerably entrenched that, even where a prominent personality is known to have died of AIDS, obituaries extolling the deceased's record of achievements do not mention the cause of death. As Nyairo writes:

The attitude many people have developed towards AIDS sufferers and their families has to do with, first, the ignorance and misinformation that many of us have about the disease, and second, the secrecy and trepidation with which victims and their families handle the affliction spread a cloak of mystery and dread around the subject of AIDS'.

(Nyairo, 1991:7)

In a society where death is a public concern, shrouding the cause of death of a prominent person implies that ordinary people too must conceal the death of their HIV-seropositive relatives. Thus concealment has been emulated by the public, and it would seem this only accentuates the problem of managing AIDS, and need for its reversal cannot be over emphasized.

Conclusions

Despite limited resources, a good deal has been achieved in the HIV/AIDS field in Kenya. Significant achievements have been made in blood screening, health education, promotion of safer sex practices, and drug research. These achievements, however, do not provide room for complacency, as no downward trend in the incidence of HIV/AIDS has yet been noticeable. The political leadership has to be more responsive and desist from cocooning itself in a culture of invulnerability, drawn from traditional ideologies which identify HIV/AIDS as a unique problem of the so-called risky groups. To be sure, HIV/AIDS threatens the entire Kenyan population, and it is ironic that, despite such a realization, not much is being done to mobilize local resources for this cause. National priorities need to be set right, and with the potential devastating consequences of HIV/AIDS to national development, it is hard to see any other priority that would rank higher, at least for now. Rhetoric may be good if it helps, but at times pragmatism and realism are better virtues. It is time that the political leadership in Kenya and elsewhere on the African continent, where HIV/AIDS is becoming endemic, took firm and decisive actions to combat this problem, making full use of local resources. If such a challenge is not to be taken seriously, and with the prospects of either a cure or vaccine for HIV/AIDS being a remote possibility, Africa may yet be slowly sinking deeper into the sea of poverty and economic degradation.

Notes

1   At the 1990 exchange rate of Kshs. 50 to one pound sterling this price equals roughly 60 pence. Since then, however, the Kenya Shilling has undergone considerable devaluation.
2   President Moi was addressing the nation during the 28th Independence Day anniversary celebrations at Nyayo Stadium, Nairobi on 12 December 1991. This was not part of his official speech, but a sudden off-the-cuff reference in his subsequent Swahili speech.

3 Dr Mboya Okeyo, Head of the National AIDS Committee, was speaking at the closing ceremony of the third annual AIDS awareness Drama and Music festival which was sponsored by the World Vision International at the Kenya Cultural Centre Nairobi.

Acknowledgement

I wish to acknowledge the financial assistance given by the International Development Research Centre of Canada, the University of London, the Overseas Research Students Award Scheme, and the University of Nairobi. However, the views expressed in this paper are strictly those of the author, and do not in any way reflect the views of any of these organizations.

References

COHEN, M. (1991) 'Changing to Safer Sex: Personality, logic and habit', in AGGLETON, P., HART, G. and DAVIES, P. (Eds) *AIDS: Responses, Interventions and Care*, London: Falmer Press.

DAWSON, J. (1991) 'Gay men's views and experiences of the HIV test', in AGGLETON, P., HART, G. and DAVIES, P. (Eds) *AIDS: Responses, Interventions and Care*, London: Falmer Press.

HOLLAND, J., RAMAZANOGLU, C., SCOTT, S. and THOMPSON, R. (1991) 'Between embarrassment and trust: Young women and diversity of condom use', in AGGLETON, P., HART, G. and DAVIES, P. (Eds) *AIDS: Responses, Interventions and Care*, London: Falmer Press.

INGHAM, R., WOODCOCK, A. and STENNER, K. (1992) 'The limitations of rational decision-making models as applied to young people's sexual behaviour', in AGGLETON, P., DAVIES, P. and HART, G. (Eds) *AIDS: Rights, Risks and Reason*, London: Falmer Press.

JACKSON, H. (1988) 'A Hidden Phenomenon', in RIEDER, I. and RUPPELT, P., *AIDS: The Woman*, San Francisco, CA: Cleis Press.

KALIBALA, S. and KALEEBA, N. (1989) 'AIDS and community-based care in Uganda: The AIDS support organisation TASO', *AIDS Care*, **1**, 2, pp. 173–7.

KIBAKI, M. (1991) 'AIDS epidemic: Situational analysis', in NJENGA, E.M. and MUITA, M. (Eds) *AIDS and the Family — Sharing the Challenges*, report of the Kenya Medical Women's Association and the Kenya National AIDS Control Programme on the first Parliamentarians Seminar on AIDS, National Assembly Buildings, Old Chambers, Nairobi, 28 November.

KIBWANA, K. (1992) *HIV/AIDS and the Law in Kenya: Preliminary Observations*, Working Paper No. 484, Institute for Development Studies, University of Nairobi.

LAVER, S.M.L. (1988) 'African communities in the struggle against AIDS: The planned for new approach', in FLEMING, A.F., CARBALLO, M., FITZSIMONS, D.W., BAILEY, M.R. and MANN, J. (Eds) *The Global Impact of AIDS*, New York, Alan Riss, Inc.

MANN, J. (1988a) 'Worldwide epidemiology of AIDS', in FLEMING, A.F., CARBALLO,

M., FITZSIMONS, D.W., BAILEY, M.R. and MANN, J. (Eds) *The Global Impact of AIDS*, New York, Alan Riss, Inc.

MANN, J. (1988b) 'Global AIDS: Epidemiology, impact, projection, global strategy, in WHO' (Ed.) *AIDS Prevention and Control*, Oxford: Pergamon Press.

MINISTRY OF HEALTH (1988) The national AIDS programme of Kenya: A five-year plan for AIDS control 1987–91, Nariobi, Ministry of Health.

MINISTRY OF HEALTH (1989) *The Republic of Kenya: Review of Kenya AIDS Control Programme*, Geneva: WHO/GPA.

MINISTRY OF HEALTH (1992a) *National AIDS Control Programme: Second Medium Term Plan 1992/1996*, WHO/GPA.

MINISTRY OF HEALTH (1992b) *National AIDS control Programme: Review 2/3/92–3/4/92*, World Health Organization/Global AIDS Programme.

MUTURI, J. and NZYUKO, S. (1988) 'National survey on the effectiveness of the radio as a means of communication: The case of AIDS programme broadcast through the Voice of Kenya', Nairobi.

MOERKERK, H. and AGGLETON, P. (1990) AIDS prevention strategies in Europe: A comparison and critical analysis', in AGGLETON, P., DAVIES, P. and HART, G. (Eds) *AIDS: Individual, Cultural and Policy Dimensions*, London: Falmer Press.

NELSON, N. (1987) 'Selling her kiosk, Kikuyu notions of sexuality and sex for sale in Mathare Valley', Kenya, in CAPLAN, P. (Ed) *The Cultural Construction of Sexuality*, London: Tavistock.

NIENGA, E.M. and MUIIA, M. (1991) (Eds) *AIDS and the Family — Sharing the Challenges*, a report of the Kenya Medical Women's Association and the Kenya National AIDS Control Programme on the first Parliamentarians Seminar on AIDS, National Assembly Buildings, Old Chambers, 28 November.

NYAIRO, J.W. (1992) 'Change this negative view of AIDS', *The Daily Nation*, 3 August.

OYOO, O. (1992a) 'AIDS: The killer not taken so seriously', *The Daily Nation*, 9 January.

OYOO, O. (1992b) 'Dissolve National AIDS Committee', *The Daily Nation*, 22 July.

PANOS DOSSIER (1990) *The Third Epidemic: Repressions of the Fear of AIDS*, London: Panos Publication.

SILVERMAN, D. (1990) 'The social organisation of HIV counselling', in AGGLETON, P., DAVIES, P. and HART, G. (Eds) *AIDS: Individual, Cultural and Policy Dimensions*, Basingstoke: Falmer Press.

The Standard (1991) December, 13, Nairobi: The Standard Newspapers.

WATNEY, S. (1991) 'AIDS: The second decade', in AGGLETON, P., HART, G. and DAVIES, P. (Eds) *AIDS: Responses, Interventions and Care*, London: Falmer Press.

WAWER, M.J., SERWADDA, D., MUSGRAVE, S.D., KONDE-LULE, J.K., MUSAGARA, M. and SEWANKAMBO, N.K. (1991) 'Dynamics of spread of HIV-1 in a rural district of Uganda', *British Medical Journal*, **303**, pp. 1303–6.

WILTON, T. and AGGLETON, P. (1991) 'Condoms, coercion and control: Heterosexuality and the limits to HIV/AIDS education', in AGGLETON, P., HART, G. and DAVIES, P. (Eds) *AIDS: Responses, Interventions and Care*, London: Falmer Press.

Chapter 13

Issues for HIV Prevention with Men who have Sex with Men: The Experience of MESMAC

Katie Deverell, Alan Prout and Tom Doyle

MESMAC (Men who have Sex with Men Action in the Community) was a three year community development project funded by the Health Education Authority (HEA). The project comprised four sites in different parts of England (London, Leicester, Leeds and Newcastle upon Tyne) which were linked together by a national structure.[1] Each site had a general brief to work with men who have sex with men (MSM) in relation to HIV/safer sex and other health needs, and a more specific brief of its own.[2]

The idea for the MESMAC project arose from a review of safer sex workshops carried out for the HEA (Gordon, 1988). This brought together empirical data from a survey of existing workshops and a theoretical framework for health promotion (French and Adams, 1986). One of the main conclusions of the review was the need to move towards a collective action model of health promotion rather than concentrating on individual behaviour change. As part of the HEA-AIDS programme, MESMAC was therefore set up to do prevention work with MSM using a community development (CD) approach.

From the outset MESMAC was working with a fundamental tension; as a CD project it was firmly rooted in the idea of working within the context of community and yet it incorporated terminology based around sexual practice, rather than identity. The group (MSM) towards whom the project was targeted was not defined in community terms at all. While it was clear that CD was at least feasible as a way of working with gay men, it was not at all clear whether or how community development might work with behaviourally defined MSM. This meant that the project was from the start involved in a complex exploration of the relationship between community, identity and behaviour.

These issues were particularly interesting given that MESMAC was an HIV project. Much organizing in the west around HIV/AIDS has arisen from within and continues to be resourced and supported by lesbian and gay communities. This has led some to argue that the response to HIV/AIDS has strengthened the lesbian and gay community, through providing it with a powerful motivating and organizing force (Altman, 1986:102; Plummer, 1988). Such community responses were necessary because at the time official institutions were unconcerned. However, in addition to this mobilizing tendency the impact of HIV can be seen to have had a more fragmenting effect, as the realities of the epidemic have highlighted the boundaries of, and diversity within, communities (Murray, 1992). This has refocused debates about identity and practice and raised questions about the inclusiveness of community. As Patton notes:

> Activists and educators, too, find themselves confronted with the disparity between notions of communities and the realities of sex and drug practices. The notion of 'community' required adherence to identity categories; yet AIDS activists were increasingly concerned to delink practices and identity, so that for example men-having-sex-with-men could recognise the risks involved without having to reorganise their identity and claim to be gay.
>
> (Patton, 1990:8)

The inclusiveness of lesbian and gay communities has also been challenged with regard to race and gender in relation to support, prevention and service provision (Patton, 1990; Altman, 1986; Dada, 1990), for example, through the neglect of the needs of Black MSM by gay community-based groups. The social response to HIV has therefore served to highlight difference and brought into focus the multiplicity of identity. This in itself can be seen to threaten the idea of community (see Patton, 1990), based as it is on the notion of commonality (Cohen, 1985).

Working within the context of HIV and being a CD project for MSM, MESMAC was clearly enmeshed in debates concerning identity, practice, community and diversity and the work continually engaged with these issues. We believe that the strength of the project lay in its ability and commitment to work with these two at times contradictory notions — building community and working with diversity. In this chapter we highlight some of what was learned through this experience, through focusing on practical examples. The aim of this is to highlight issues which may be of interest to others undertaking similar work. Through this, we also hope to raise questions about community, identity and sexuality (for a further discussion of these issues see Prout and Deverell, 1994). First we will begin with a description of the background to MESMAC, situating it in the wider context of work with MSM, and providing a brief exploration of the community development approach.

Katie Deverell, Alan Prout and Tom Doyle

Background to MESMAC

MESMAC was a product of what might be described as the second phase of the social reaction to the HIV epidemic in Britain. The first phase, which ended around 1987, has been well documented (see, for example, Weatherburn, *et al.*, 1992; and Weeks, 1989) and we will not repeat this except to say that it had two features. On the one hand there was a widespread (and continuing) fear and prejudice about AIDS which found expression in both unofficial circles (for example in media coverage) and in official indifference at a policy level. This phase was well characterized by Patton (1985) as one of homophobia, sexophobia and germophobia. On the other hand was the grassroots response of gay communities and other AIDS activists who began, in the face of governmental inaction, to build support and care systems and organize preventive education (King, 1993). By the mid-1980s, links had been formed with sections of the health professions and influential policy advisers and this alliance was, by 1987, able to establish AIDS an important matter for public health policy (Berridge, 1992).

MESMAC was part of this policy response. The HEA assumed its remit for AIDS Public Education work near the end of 1987. The years of official inaction had, however, left a legacy of mistrust especially among AIDS activists, gay communities, HIV/AIDS voluntary organizations and ethnic minority groups. The contemporary government's mass media campaign was criticized for its emphasis on scare tactics, its moralizing undertones and the inaccuracy of some of its messages (Watney, 1987, 1988; Carter and Watney, 1989). There was a sense that the health propaganda of the time was motivated primarily by a concern that HIV might spread to the general population and in this sense continued the homophobic prejudice of the earlier period. The HEA's work up until this point was thought by many activists to have suffered from the effects of this general climate. In particular, there were many demands that the absence of a prevention programme for gay men be remedied. Partly in response to these pressures the HEA set up, using the then fashionable terminology, a Men Who Have Sex with Men (MSM) Programme. MESMAC was one important part of this programme, and was one of the first attempts to bridge the gap between governmental institutions and community-based gay and HIV/AIDS organizations.

At the time that MESMAC started there was very little work occurring specifically for MSM in Britain. As King (1993), Rooney and Scott (1992) and McKevitt, Warwick and Aggleton (1994) have documented, for a variety of reasons the early work begun by gay men around HIV and safer sex in the eighties had in many cases not continued. With the emphasis on targeting the general population, this meant that the needs of MSM were neglected by both the voluntary and statutory sector. MESMAC was one of the few projects set up to meet the needs of MSM, including gay and bisexual men, although its MSM title meant that this was not always recognized. This meant that a lot of the work undertaken by the MESMAC projects involved building up local infra-structures, developing resources and lobbying for organizational and policy support to do work with MSM.

The community development philosophy of MESMAC impacted greatly on the project and affected the way the work was done. As far as we know it was the first statutorily funded project explicitly to adopt a community development approach to HIV work with MSM. In many ways, the project was therefore breaking new ground, although where possible the workers did try to build on any work that was already taking place. The CD focus marked off the work of the project from much of the other work that was occurring. As King, Rooney and Scott (1992) found in a survey of UK initiatives targeting work at gay and bisexual men, of the few initiatives that existed most were public education events and outreach. Whilst MESMAC also undertook this type of work, the CD philosophy in the project meant that lobbying, collective work and organizational development were also prioritized. By the time the HEA funding for the project ended, a push at national and regional level for MSM work as well as local lobbying had led to an increase in the number of gay men's/MSM projects in Britain. By the end of January, 1993, for example, McKevitt, Warwick and Aggleton (1994) found that out of 49 projects set up for MSM, 15 were using a community-based approach or had a strong degree of community involvement. In these changing circumstances the MESMAC workers found themselves with an important role to play in training and networking with new workers.

MESMAC and Community Development

As noted above, one of the crucial factors in enabling the MESMAC workers to combine the benefits of community-based work with the importance of recogniz-ing diversity was the CD strategy and theoretical principles which guided the work. There are several different definitions of community development (see for example, Martin, 1990; Smithies, 1991; Sheffield Health Authority, 1993). Rather than something that can be given a water-tight definition, CD is perhaps best seen as a way of working, informed by certain principles, which encourages people to identify common concerns and which supports them in taking action related to them. When MESMAC was established, the HEA's own definition included the following principles of working: i) working with groups rather than individuals; ii) prioritizing disadvantaged and marginalized groups; iii) encour-aging a positive holistic view of health; iv) aiming to increase self-confidence; v) aiming to improve relationships between professionals and voluntary and statutory groups although it may also challenge statutory organizations to meet needs; vi) (the community) defining its own needs, rather than receiving a professionally presented list of needs; vii) seeing work as important in its own right and; and viii) valuing people whatever their background, starting from where they are, and challenging discriminatory or oppressive behaviour from individuals or bureaucracies and (ix) promoting access to information and resources (Smithies and Adams, 1990).

In the post-war period, community development occupies and has constructed ways of handling the space between 'bottom-up', autonomous, grassroots activities and 'top-down' initiatives from both government and voluntary organizations. To the grassroots, it promises a way of influencing official attitudes and policies and access to public resources; to officialdom it presents ways of relating more effectively and realistically with difficult client groups and hitherto intractable social problems, as well as a route to public participation and meeting consumer need, notions which emerged as powerful themes in the social policy of the 1980s. To some extent this explains why the form of collective action which MESMAC took was that of community development. However, CD is not the only form of collective action (Homans and Aggleton, 1998). Overtly political groups in the HIV field such as ACT-UP are also based in the grassroots and take collective action. Such groups tend to be oppositional to government and other official institutions such as the pharmaceutical industry. They have been able to collectivize action in the form of radical political protest and calls for sweeping social changes. Because CD occupies a more ambivalent position, somewhere between government and communities, it offers a different way of working, with social change achieved through more domesticated means. It does not, for example, eschew campaigns to change service provision, but tends to advocate less dramatic forms of protest (such as lobbying or winning representation in the decision-making of statutory organizations). To say this is to criticize neither form of collective action, but it is to recognize their rather different positions in the field of action. Because MESMAC brought together a range of different people and organizations (a government agency, freelance professionals, statutory and voluntary sector organizations, front-line workers who identified with gay and black communities, and academic researchers), CD was an appropriate way of working to adopt.

It is important at this point to distinguish community development from community-based work, of which there are many varieties. Community-based outreach, for example, has been increasingly used in relation to HIV, especially when particular groups, for example, drug users, are seen as vulnerable but hard to reach. Work is initiated which aims to reach individuals outside the formal setting of an agency (a clinic, for example) by contacting people in the settings of their everyday life. Workers might contact people on the streets, or in pubs and cafes, or a housing estate, or in prisons, hostels or youth clubs. When contact has been made it might be followed up by providing individuals with health information or other resources (such as condoms or syringe cleansing equipment) and trying to attract them into the services that are available.

One key difference between this sort of work and community development is that CD aims to work collectively rather than with individuals. CD may start

Grass roots Work	*Participation Strategy*
e.g. Outreach	e.g. Lobbying
Starting new groups	Policy Work
Building Community Infrastructure	*Organizational Development*
e.g. Establishing networks	e.g. Involving users in steering groups
Resourcing existing groups	Establishing advisory groups

Figure 13.1   The CD strategy used by MESMAC

with individuals but it aims at helping individuals to group together to take collective action. Another difference is that it is prepared to take on changing social conditions and services if that is what is seen by groups and communities to be appropriate.

Understanding of the CD approach within MESMAC took some time, but the project has shown that it can be successfully translated into practice by front-line workers who have no special experience or background in it. Three factors seem important: first, that the workers have an understanding of the communities themselves and groups they work with (most directly by being members themselves) or are in a position to develop it. Second, that appropriate training and support are provided. Third, that the theory of community development be available in a coherent and comprehensible way which can be readily related to practical experience.

The strategy used by MESMAC stressed the need to work at several different levels (see Figure 13.1): Grass roots work, to build on shared experiences and promote new solutions to locally defined problems and issues; building community infrastructure by bringing individuals and groups together; organizational development to encourage organizations to change in response to identified needs; and participation, finding ways to involve MSM in the project, particularly its decision-making processes (Figure 13.1).

Underlying this strategy were important CD principles relating to points such as working from established need, encouraging consultation and participation and having a commitment to equal opportunities. Above all the CD approach was about working collectively in a way that encourages a holistic view of health, rather than focusing purely on individual behaviour change (see Webster, 1991). The key to the success of the CD strategy was the direct contact, flexibility and responsiveness it engendered. Projects were able to be very flexible about the methods and areas of work they established as long as they could integrate them into the CD strategy. By the end of the HEA funding period, the project as a whole had undertaken 91 different initiatives (Figure 13.2).

Fifteen initiatives involved outreach and/or work with individuals. For example:
* streetwork in public sex environments;
* one-to-one telephone advice and counselling;
* outreach with black MSM using saunas;
* outreach work on the commercial gay scene;
* work with gay men on an inner-city housing estate.

Thirty-one initiatives involved work with existing organizations. For example:
* lobbying, liaison and strategy development for more and better statutory sector HIV prevention for MSM;
* development, fund raising and training for black gay and lesbian helpline;
* networks and forums for HIV/AIDS gay and lesbian workers (including one specifically for black workers);
* a small grants scheme for individuals and voluntary organizations wishing to develop initiatives for MSM;
* work for and with educational organizations (including schools, colleges and universities).

Twenty-three new groups have been set up (either by MSM alone or in collaboration with others). For example:
* Latex Productions (a Lesbian and Gay Theatre Group);
* Rent Boy Action (a self-help group for male prostitutes);
* a Police Monitoring Group;
* Gay Men's Health Groups;
* a Young Men's Peer Training Group;
* Young Gay Men's Groups;
* Black Gay Groups (for young and older men);
* a Black Peer Training Project;
* Gay Men Tyneside (providing social alternatives to the commercial scene and other activities including safer sex education);
* Pink Ink (a group producing a gay and lesbian newspaper);
* a Gay Men's Photography Group;
* a Married Men's Group.

Twenty-two other diverse initiatives have been undertaken. For example:
* a condom distribution scheme in gay pubs and clubs;
* leaflet, poster and other materials tailored to particular localities and target groups;
* safer sex workshops for various target groups;
* health and beauty workshops for black men;
* developing a safer sex pack for men with learning difficulties.

Figure 13.2   Initiatives undertaken by MESMAC 1990–1993

This involved making contact with 7500 users on just under 20 000 different occasions. In addition, all of the local projects carried out a great deal of work with or in relation to other organizations in the voluntary and statutory sector, overall there was contact with at least 3185 other workers. MESMAC found that grassroots work can be connected with correcting community resources for meeting HIV-related need, and improving services provided by both the voluntary and statutory sector (for a more detailed discussion see Prout and Deverell, 1992; Prout and Deverell, 1994).

Having briefly described the background to the project, we now discuss some of the practically based learning around the themes of community, identity and diversity.

Building on and Building up Community

One of the key principles that informed the development of MESMAC was that it should draw on and recognize the existing grassroots work which had taken place within gay communities around HIV and safer sex. This idea was put into practice early on through an initial forum where representatives from lesbian and gay, and IIIV organizations were involved in developing and discussing the MESMAC project proposal. Such involvement was carried through into the writing of the site proposals; this ethic of consultation and participation was continued throughout the project. All the workers spent time establishing what was already taking place within their local community in order to consult and find out needs, and to build on, learn from and integrate MESMAC initiatives with existing work. Contrary to some suggestions (see Scott, 1993) the term MSM did not seem to alienate the voluntary sector, all the sites worked successfully with a large number of lesbian, gay and bisexual groups. This took the form of needs assessment; joint work; resourcing existing gay groups; providing resources to develop new groups; providing training and support; and networking.

In this respect, the experiences of Leicester MESMAC as a black project were somewhat different. They found that there were hardly any black community groups in Leicester which formed around a specific sexual identity so there were few existing resources to draw on. Indeed the MESMAC experience shows that specific efforts are needed to contact black MSM and it cannot be assumed that black men will be reached through general MSM or gay men's work. In fact the Leicester project found that much of its work involved thinking about and trying to create a specifically black gay culture rather than expecting black men to fit into European ideas of gay identity and culture. However, they did work with existing groups, both through supporting and networking with other black groups, and through working to get the needs of black MSM incorporated into existing lesbian and gay organizations.

One of the advantages of working with gay communities was the ability to target existing networks of gay and bisexual men through community organizations, networks and meeting places. For example, one of the important focuses for all the sites was the local gay scene which proved to be a good place to reach large numbers of white gay men. The projects also used the gay press and other community networks to advertise MESMAC initiatives and feed back information. Where such local networks were not well developed, MESMAC helped build them up. One way was through the development of Pink Ink (a lesbian and gay freesheet) in Leeds. Such work enabled projects to build up their image as part of the local gay community and contributed to building community infrastructure.

Through working with existing community organisations, the workers were also able to draw on local experiences of lesbian and gay groups. Many existing organizations had a history of using shared experience and support as a base, both in relation to political action and service provision. This was something the workers were able to learn from and develop through building on gay men's sense of community and finding ways to relate this to safer sex and HIV. Working with existing networks of gay and bisexual men also had the advantage of informing workers about other networks. Combined with their own knowledge of local communities the workers were able to use this information to target other places where men met, such as local public sex environments.

Although using existing networks was crucial, particularly in contacting gay and bisexual men, it also had limitations. For example, the workers found that many young gay men do not read the gay press, use scene venues, or take part in gay cultural or political movements; this was also true of many black men. As many gay-identified men were not linked into gay community organizations, further effort was needed to target them. Often this involved setting up new initiatives to meet their needs.

Working through gay-identified networks also did not reach non-gay identifying men who have sex with men. Contact with these men in other settings reinforced the view that many of them felt isolated from the gay community. Thus it was important to find other ways to meet these men. The workers found that outreach, one to one work, phone work, encouraging referrals from other organizations, advertising in the general press, specific group work, and non-identifying leaflets were all good ways to reach MSM, as was working with others to incorporate the needs of MSM into generic work. MESMAC experience shows that work with existing gay and bisexual communities is a good focal point and it is important for projects to draw on the skills and experiences of men here. Often there is a history of lesbian and gay organizing which can be built on. However, it is also important to work outside gay-identified networks and find other ways to contact non-identifying MSM.

Identity, Community and Collective Action

One of the early experiences of the project was that it was easier to work collectively with men who had open and confident gay identities (c.f. Davis *et al.*, 1991). Workers found it particularly hard to collectivize work with men who did not identify as gay or bisexual or who wanted to keep their sexual identity secret. It is instructive in this respect that Patton, describing the work of John D'Emilio, Jeffrey Weeks and Michael Bronski in relation to the development of modern gay identities and community, notes that, 'Each views the development of a public sexual identification as a key stage in the process of identity and community formation' (Patton, 1985:123). Indeed, MESMAC workers found that it was much easier to develop collective action with those men who were willing to be out about their sexual identity. This underlines an important difference with much other CD work which is organized around identities, issues or communities that are public, or that people are happy to be associated with (for example, their place of residence). Many MSM do not have a public sexual identity, or indeed do not want an identity based around their sexual practice. This makes immediate collective action more difficult as work usually has to proceed in ways that will not publicly identify them. This obviously limits the kind of activities that can be undertaken.

The workers found that many MSM who did not identify as gay were resistant to the forms of collective action they attempted, and were only interested in accessing resources and information. One of the main reasons for this was that for many men having sex with other men was something that they kept secret. For these men working collectively meant the risk of their being identified as a MSM or being open about their activities in a way that was totally unacceptable and unrealistic. In any case, for many men having sex with other men was all that they wanted, they did not see themselves as part of a community and felt they had little in common with others with whom they had sex. It was important that this was respected and that it was not assumed that all MSM wanted to come out and adopt a gay identity (see also Bartos, McLeod and Nott, 1993; Prestage and Hood, 1993). For example, many of the black men in the Leicester project met in saunas and made a distinction between themselves as MSM and gay men with whom they did not identify (see Deverell, 1992). For these men the value of the project lay in the opportunity to access resources without having to identify as gay or bisexual.

Within MESMAC it did prove possible, if done sensitively, to form groups for (or including) non-gay-identified men, by focusing around other issues. For example, Rent Boy Action in Leeds (a self-help group for young men selling sex) was focused around legal rights and dealing with harassment. This work involved such things as building up trust in order to find out men's needs and developing groups around these and the use of non-gay identifying venues and strict confidentiality. Workers also encouraged individual men to get involved in particular groups of interest to them.

Although it was recognized that collective action was not always appropriate in relation to non-identifying MSM (outreach, phone work and one-to-one work being preferable) — for some men this was important. For those who wanted it, the opportunity to meet, talk with and get support from other men in a similar situation was very valuable, particularly in reducing isolation and reassuring men that others were in a similar situation.

For those men who had a sexual identity, and who were open about it, collective work was significantly easier. This was often the case as many gay-identified men became involved as a way to support other gay men, or to share their experiences with others. Through the process of sharing experiences and working collectively, being put in touch with other groups and organizations, making new friends and being able to develop their own initiatives, many of those who became involved felt a strengthened sense of community. For some men, contact with the project led to a greater certainty and confidence in their own sexual identity which led to a decision to come out. This way of working also showed evidence of men adopting and maintaining safer sex, through promoting self esteem and strengthening attachment to the gay community and gay identity (see also Kippax *et al.*, 1990; King, 1993). Working from a basis of existing community organisation and shared identity was therefore very helpful in collectivizing work with gay and bisexual men. Although it should be noted that not all gay men wanted to attend groups and those who were not out, or just coming out could find the prospect of going to a gay group intimidating.

Although the MESMAC experience shows that it is much easier to attract men to groups if they share something in common, this 'thing' may be additional to their sexuality. Often sexual identity is not enough, or rather other differences are more important than a shared sexual identity. Some of the most long-running MESMAC groups were those based on specific activities which were additional to gay identity and provided an organizing focus, for example, Latex Productions, a lesbian and gay theatre group. This does not mean that sexual identity is not important, but on its own it is not always sufficient as a focus for organization. Other differences and experiences such as class, race or political views can fracture any unity based on shared sexual identity. Within MESMAC recognition of this diversity and complexity highlighted the limitations of using categories based on identity.

Multiplicity of Identity

Another of the important practical experiences in the work was the need to recognize that men may have more than one identity, and attachment to various communities. In particular, the work with black men highlighted the need for a more complex understanding of the interplay of race and sexuality on people's identities. For some men their sexual identity is not always the most important or prominent identity. For example, living in a racist society, many black men experience a greater need for social support around race than sexuality. This is particularly the case since black men are more likely to be identified and discriminated against on the basis of race. This means that many black MSM are more likely to get involved in, and take action around, the social and political issues affecting black communities, rather than organize around sexuality.

This situation was not unique to black men. Many of the issues also arose in MESMAC work with South East Asian and Jewish men. It was also true of white men. For example, at times their age, class or occupation could be more important than their sexual identity. MESMAC has shown that people have different identities which are more or less important in relation to different situations, times and people (see also Gatter, 1991, 1993; Weeks, 1990). The importance of considering the multiplicity of identity should, however, not be seen in a simplistic way. As Avtar Brah has written,

> Structures of class, racism, gender and sexuality cannot be treated as 'independent variables' because the oppression of each is inscribed within the other — is constituted by and is constitutive of the other.
>
> (Brah, 1992:137)

Thus it is not simply a case of thinking about race and thinking about sexuality and trying to fit these issues together, but considering how race and sexuality interact and affect each other, e.g. in terms of the way ideas about race construct Black men's sexuality as exotic and animalistic (Manuel, Fani-Koyode and Gupta 1989; see also Brake, 1976 on gender and sexuality).

The multiplicity of identity underlines another important point, that gay men themselves have different understandings of the notion of a gay identity and do not attach equal importance to it. For example, some men though identifying as gay do not feel that they have a lot in common with other gay men. This means that sexual identity has different meanings for people and as such it is not necessarily a unifying factor.[3]

Who to work with?

At the time the project was set up, the use of the term MSM was in vogue, its importance being seen to lie in the fact that it recognized that there is no necessary link between identity and behaviour. However, as the project developed the term came under criticism (see for example, Watney, 1993). One of the criticisms stated that,

> Conceptualisation of the work based on MSM model tends to lead to an emphasis upon targeting men on the margins at the expense of men at the core of the gay and bisexual communities.
>
> (Scott, 1993: Appendix 1)

At first sight such a reading of the term may seem convincing, and indeed in the very early days of the project some of the workers thought they should prioritize work with non-gay identified men. However, this perception soon changed and often project members would describe the project as gay men's work. This no doubt reflects the fact that the vast majority of those reached by MESMAC were gay identified men (80–85 per cent). One of the important experiences of MESMAC is that having a brief related to working with MSM does not mean that the needs of gay and bisexual men are neglected. However, it did mean that there was a commitment to meet the needs of all MSM through finding ways also to reach more marginalized men. The fact that the CD strategy emphasized the importance of working around the basis of expressed need gave the workers particular flexibility in this area, since it legitimized the development of specific initiatives for men who identified in different ways.

The experience of MESMAC is that MSM are a diverse group, and there is not clear relationship between sexual identity and practice. For example, some men were very out and identified as gay or bisexual; others identified as gay or bisexual but were not out; others did not have a definite sexual identity; still others did not feel a need to have a sexual identity or felt the identities available to them were not culturally appropriate. Even if people did have a clear sexual identity, this was not always revealing about sexual behaviour. For example, men identifying as gay may be having sex with women, and men who identified as straight would be having sex with men. This complex situation reinforced the lack of necessary commensurability between identity and practice which is well documented in sexuality and sex research literature (Boulton and Weatherburn, 1990; Davies, 1990; Davis *et al.*, 1991; Weatherburn *et al.*, 1992; British Market Research Bureau, Ltd (BMRB) 1992; Siegal and Bauman, 1986). Therefore, trying to consider the fluidity of sexuality using categories based on identity had limitations.

Debates about the best concepts to use continued throughout the life of the project. MSM was seen to be useful because it recognized the diversity and fluidity of sexuality and encouraged workers to think about non-gay-identified men. However, it was felt by some to deny the history and culture of gay men, and to neglect gay men's attachment to identity. Politically, workers also wanted to highlight work with gay men and get their needs recognized. Given the importance of working with as wide a range of men as possible, MSM was felt to be the best option. There was a concern that people would not make the extra effort to target non-gay- identifying men if projects were defined in terms of gay and bisexual men. This was particularly important in relation to black men, as the MESMAC experience indicated that most black MSM do not relate to HIV prevention that is organized around gay identity. However, it was recognized that there were not clear cut answers, both concepts had benefits and drawbacks, the terms gay and bisexual may attract some men but would clearly alienate others.

Who does the Work?

Most of the workers in the project were gay-identified men and this proved to be a great asset in the development of the work, with many gay-identified users commenting that it helped to build trust as well as provide a feeling of empathy and understanding. Although it was felt best to have gay men work with other gay men, it was important to recognize that being gay did not necessarily mean that workers would have had similar experiences with users, for example, sometimes other differences such as class meant that they had very different life experiences and lifestyles. There was also an issue about whether gay workers were best to work with non-gay-identified men. For example, because of their own strong gay identity, a difficulty for some of the workers was in accepting that not all MSM wanted to identify as gay. Many of the workers wanted to support men coming out and validate their gay identity (see also Davis, 1991) however, as the work progressed they realized that the situation was more complex. Many of the MSM did not see themselves as gay, or did not want to take on this identity. The workers felt that as very out gay men they may alienate some men who have sex with men.

An important related point was the need to consider whether all jobs including administration and support roles need to be held by MSM. The project's experience is that given appropriate skills and sensitivity, they need not, but that such workers need appropriate support.

One of the benefits of being part of the community was that the workers became known and trusted and were often able to build up informal links which were useful in the work. However, a difficulty in this respect was that living and working in the same community and having a code of conduct which stressed the importance of sexual boundaries, meant that the work had an impact on the workers' own social and sexual life (see Deverell, 1993 for a discussion of these issues).

In relation to workers being part of the communities with whom they worked, a further issue arose involving black men. The workers found that some men did not identify themselves as black, or felt they had little in common with other black men and therefore actually preferred to talk to white workers. Some black men were also in relationships with white partners and worried about alienating them through becoming involved in a black project. This situation was made more difficult since the workers found that by concentrating their efforts on targeting black men, many assumed that the project was political rather than there to provide a service. As a worker explained, 'Because you have "Black" in your title, you become a pressure group rather than a service provider.'

The workers felt that black men sometimes shied away from contact with the project because of this. For others there was a fear of being identified as a MSM. This meant that some men felt threatened by the approach of someone from the same community. This meant that some black men actually preferred to talk to white workers. This underlines the importance of not making assumptions as to how people choose to identify themselves, or with whom they will feel most comfortable.

Who is in the Community

One of the issues in working from a basis of existing community organization involved who was defined as belonging to the community. Not all gay-identified men were seen to be part of the community, or felt excluded from it. For example, some of the gay-identified rent boys said that many gay men looked down upon them, or made it clear that they did not want rent boys associated with the gay community. Thus not all self-identified gay men were seen to be part of the community and some felt excluded by it. Organizing work around identity and community therefore could have the disadvantage of reproducing existing inequalities related to race, ability, class and age. This is an issue that has been pointed out by other commentators in relation to earlier grassroots work around safer sex (Patton, 1990; Dada, 1990; Altman, 1988), and is supported by the MESMAC experience. For example deaf gay men and black gay men contacted by the project have argued very strongly that they have missed out on previous information and support, or that available services, information and support have been inappropriate or inaccessible.

The importance of equal opportunities within the CD approach meant that the projects had a commitment to make their initiatives as accessible as possible. They did this through such things as providing signers, child care, subsidising events, having black-only events, free food, and through challenging racism and sexism within groups. Through this the projects were particularly successful in attracting men who had previously felt isolated or marginalized from gay communities, and enabled them to feel part of a community. Many of those involved in MESMAC initiatives said that they had valued the opportunity to meet men they would never have met socially, and to have been made to think about issues relating to black men, deaf men and working men. This underlines the diversity of experience amongst men who identify as gay or bisexual and the need for workers to consider who is included and who left out in the existing communities they choose to work with.

Work with Women

Orienting work around gay identity and community obviously had benefits, but it could have the effect of silencing certain issues or making them difficult to address, for example through marginalizing women and men's relationships with women.[4] In the case of MESMAC, this meant that many of the gay workers found it difficult to address needs in relation to the sex men were having with women, and that at times the women working in the project felt marginalized or found it hard to raise issues relating to gender (see Deverell and Bell, 1993).

For those MSM who were having sex with women, organizing work around gay communities and identities had the effect of addressing only part of their sexuality. For example, many of the men with female partners did not know about HIV transmission routes between men and women, and having information which only addressed sex with men did not help this situation. As an HIV project, it was important that such issues were addressed, particularly as these were often of major concern to the men themselves — for example, men wanted help in negotiating safer sex with female partners, or in getting support to come out to them. It was important not to assume that such issues only applied to men who identified as straight or bisexual, as gay men may also be having sex with women (see for example, Weatherburn *et al.*, 1992; BMRB, 1992:6) a point which some commentators seem to overlook (Scott, 1993).

The experience of MESMAC shows that some work with women is important, even in a men's project. This may be through joint lobbying and support work with lesbians around issues relating to sexuality and service provision, as well as work involving sex that men may be having with women.

Varying Needs

It was thought from the start of the project that MSM may have different needs, through having different sexual identities as well as class, race or other factors. The benefit of the CD strategy in this respect was its stress on working from a basis of established need. This meant that work was organized around discovering what men actually wanted rather than making assumptions about their needs. Therefore, needs assessment in MESMAC was integral to the whole approach to work and not a one-off exercise. By monitoring, discussing and reviewing their work, the sites engaged in a process of continually developing understanding about the needs of those with whom they were working. Key to this process were a great deal of *direct* contact with MSM; flexible front line workers to respond to the emerging and changing picture of needs, autonomy to translate these directly into new initiatives; and skilful and sensitive workers, including their own experience and involvement as gay men. Identifying needs was a complex and interpretive process not a simple and mechanical one. The workers had to listen and learn and have flexibility to be responsive to both individual and local variation.

Although there were some common general needs, the MESMAC experience was that the needs of MSM were very diverse. Men who have sex with men come from a variety of class, ethnic and religious backgrounds, have different abilities and identities and different ideas about their sexuality. Because of different social and economic circumstances, not all men have the same choices or means to realize their choices; for example, MESMAC found that young men, married men, sex workers, men with learning difficulties, men who have been sexually abused, and deaf men all have particular and different needs (see also Davis *et al.*, 1991; Connell, *et al.*, 1991). Because the needs of MSM are complex and at times contradictory and there is no one right way of working, work with MSM needs to start from men's felt needs and requires a diversity of initiatives, materials and resources.

One of the continual findings of the various needs assessments was that for many men HIV is not their main priority (see also McKevitt, Warwick and Aggleton, 1994; Kjeldsen, 1991). In this respect the advantage of the CD approach was that it focused work on the issues of importance to men themselves, and therefore legitimized work which directly addressed this wider context. This meant that MESMAC work involved meeting needs related to issues such as coming out, dealing with homophobia, finding housing, in establishing social alternatives to the commercial scene and in getting legal advice and medical treatment. In this way, MESMAC did not reduce the needs of MSM to those solely concerned with HIV and other STDs. This in itself was important as MESMAC has confirmed that HIV-prevention and sexuality work cannot be separated from wider social, cultural and economic issues. For example, men may not be able to afford condoms, or men may be made homeless through coming out. Health education and promotion must engage with these issues.

Conclusion

Working within a CD strategy, MESMAC had the ability and commitment to combine both the benefits of community-based work with the importance of recognizing and addressing diversity. By developing work around sexual identity and community, the projects worked successfully with existing community organizations and networks of gay and bisexual men. Building on this basis of shared experience and support proved particularly useful in collectivizing work. However, the work also showed a diversity of need and experience amongst MSM, both within gay and bisexual communities, as well as amongst men who did not identify in this way. This highlighted how an emphasis on community and commonality can also hide diversity. The experience of MESMAC is that there is a need to look beyond the boundaries of existing communities in order to reach MSM who do not identify as gay or who feel marginalized from gay communities, because of their age, race or differing commitment to a gay identity. In this case successful collective work often involves organizing around something other than sexual identity, and recognizing the diversity of men's identities.

MESMAC has shown that *both* work based on sexual identity and work based on sexual behaviour can exclude some men and the full range of MSM will only be reached if both approaches are used. The experience of the project was that a CD strategy provides both the flexibility and the autonomy to work successfully with this diversity.

Notes

1 At the time of writing three of the four sites have successfully attracted regional funding to continue the work, the fourth is in negotiation.
2 For example, Leicester worked with black men. London worked with young men, but within that specifically targeted black MSM.
3 It is important that this is not seen simplistically. The workers found that an important consideration in relation to work with black men was to recognize that people may choose to identify themselves in different ways (see also Peterson, 1992). For example, some men felt there was a need for more black men to come out and identify as gay, and for there to be greater visibility of black, gay role models. However, others questioned the need for a gay identity which they saw as a white, western one. A lot of black MSM do not define as gay or want to. There is therefore a need to support black MSM who do not want to take on a gay identity, as well as those who chose to identify as gay.
4 Similar points have been made before by bisexual men (see George *et al.*, 1993).

Acknowledgement

We would like to thank everyone involved in the MESMAC project.

References

ALTMAN, D. (1986) *AIDS and the New Puritanism*, London: Pluto Press.
ALTMAN, D. (1988) 'Legitimation through disaster: AIDS and the gay movement', in FEE, E. and FOX, D. (Eds) *AIDS and the Burdens of History*, Berkeley and London, University of California Press.
BARTOS, M. MCLFOD, I., NOTT, P. (1993) *Meanings of Sex Between Men*, a study conducted by the Australian Federation of AIDS Organisations for the Commonwealth Department of Health, Housing, Local Government and Community Services.

BERRIDGE, V. (1992) 'AIDS: History and contemporary history', in HERDT, G. and LINDENBAUM, S. (Eds.) *The Time of AIDS: Social Analysis, Theory and Method*, London: Sage.

BOULTON, M. and WEATHERBURN, P. (1990) *Literature Review on Bisexuality and HIV Transmission*, London: Academic Department of Public Health, St. Mary's Medical School (mimeo).

BRAH, A. (1992) 'Difference, diversity and differentiation', in DONALD, J. and RATTANSI, A. (Eds) *Race, Culture and Difference*, London: Sage.

BRAKE, M. (1976) 'I may be a Queer, but at least I am a man: male hegemony and ascribed versus achieved gender', in BARKER, D. and ALLEN, S. (Eds) *Sexual Divisions and Society: Process and Change*, London: Tavistock.

BRITISH MARKET RESEARCH BUREAU LTD. (1992) *Gay Pubs and Clubs 1992, Report on a Quantitative Survey*, London, BMRB (mimeo).

CARTER, E. and WATNEY, S. (Eds) (1989) *Taking Liberties: AIDS and Cultural Politics*, London: Serpent's Tail.

CONNELL, R.W. DOWSETT, G.W., RODDEN, P., DAVIS, M.D., WATSON, L. and BAXTER, D. (1991) 'Social class, gay men and AIDS prevention', *Australian Journal of Public Health*, **15**, 3, pp. 178–89.

COHEN, A. (1985) *The Symbolic Construction of Community*, London: Ellis, Horwood and Tavistock.

DADA, M. (1990) 'Race and the AIDS agenda', in BOFFIN, T. and GUPTA, S. (Eds) *Ecstatic Antibodies: Revisiting the AIDS Mythology*, London: Rivers Oram.

DAVIES, P.M. (1990) Some Problems in Defining and Sampling Non-heterosexual Males, Project SIGMA Working Paper No. 3, London: South Bank Polytechnic.

DAVIS, M.D., KLEMMER, U. and DOWSETT, G.W. (1991) *Bisexually Active Men and Beats: Theoretical and Educational Implications*, Sydney: AIDS Council for New South Wales and Macquarie University AIDS Research Unit.

DEVERELL, K. (1992) *Outreach Work in Saunas: The Experience of Liecester Black MESMAC*, MESMAC Evaluation Working Paper No. 4, Keele University, Department of Sociology and Social Anthropology (mimeo).

DEVERELL, K. (1993) 'Out of bounds — constructing sexual boundaries at work', paper presented at ASA Conference July, Keele University, Department of Sociology and Social Anthropology (mimeo).

DEVERELL, K. and BELL, J. (1993) *Some Thoughts on Being Straight Women in a Men who have Sex with Men Project*, Keele University, Department of Sociology and Social Anthropology (mimeo).

FRENCH, J. and ADAMS, L. (1986) 'From analysis to synthesis, theories of health education', *Health Education Journal*, **45**, 2, pp. 71–4.

GATTER, P. (1991) *On Neutral Ground? The culture of HIV/AIDS voluntary organisations in London*, London: South Bank Polytechnic.

GATTER, P. (1993) 'Anthropology and the culture of HIV/AIDS voluntary organisations', in AGGLETON, P., DAVIES, P. and HART, G. (Eds) *AIDS: Facing the Second Decade*, London: Falmer Press.

GEORGE, S., DEYNEM, H., FARQUHARSON, P., WILLIAMS, G., BARKLE, D. and KIPPAX, S. (1993) *Bisexuality and HIV Prevention*, London: Health Education Authority.

GORDON, P. (1988) *Safer Sex Workshops for Gay and Bisexual Men: A Review*, London: Health Education Authority.

HOMANS, H. and AGGLETON, P. (1988) 'Health education, HIV infection and AIDS', in AGGLETON, P. and HOMANS, H. (Eds) *Social Aspects of AIDS*, Lewes: Falmer Press.

KING, E. (1993) *Safety in Numbers*, London: Cassell.

KING, E., ROONEY, M. and SCOTT, P. (1992) *HIV Prevention for Gay Men: A Survey of Initiatives in the UK*, London: North West Thames Regional Health Authority.

KIPPAX, S. *et al.* (1990) *The Importance of Gay Community in the Prevention of HIV Transmission*, Social Aspects of the Prevention of AIDS Study A, Report No. 7, Sydney, Macquarie University.

KJELDSEN, M. (1991) *Streetwise Youth Report*, London: Streetwise Youth Project.

MANUEL, P., FANI-KOYODE, R. and GUPTA, S. (1989) (Eds) 'Imaging black sexuality', in REEVES, M. and HAMMOND, J. (Eds) *Looking Beyond the Frame: Racism, Representation and Resistance*, Links 34, Oxford: Third World First.

MARTIN, R. (1990) *Definitions of Community Work*, London: Federation of Community Work Training Groups.

McKEVITT, C., WARWICK, I. and AGGLETON, P.J. (1994) *Towards Good Practice: HIV Prevention with Gay, Bisexual and Other Men who have Sex with Men*, London: HEA.

MURRAY, S.O. (1992) 'Components of gay Community in San Francisco', in HERDT, G. (Ed.) *Gay Culture in America: Essays from the Field*, Boston: Beacon Press.

PATTON, C. (1985) *Sex and Germs — the politics of AIDS*, Boston: South End Press.

PATTON, C. (1990) *Inventing AIDS*, London: Routledge.

PETERSON, J.L. (1992) 'Black men and their same-sex desires and behaviors', in HERDT, G. (Ed.) *Gay Culture in America: Essays from the Field*, Boston: Beacon Press.

PLUMMER, K. (1988) 'Organizing AIDS', in AGGLETON, P. and HOMANS, H. (Eds) *Social Aspects of AIDS*, Lewes: Falmer Press.

PRESTAGE, G. and HOOD, D. (1993) 'Targeting non-gay attached men who have sex with men: New data', outreach and cultural issues, paper given at the 7th Social Aspects of AIDS Conference, London.

PROUT, A. and DEVERELL, K. (1992) *The Impact of the MESMAC Project: An Interim Review*, MESMAC Evaluation Working Paper No. 5, Keele University, Department of Sociology and Social Anthropology (mimeo).

PROUT, A. and DEVERELL, K. (1994) *Building Community: Working with Diversity, An Evaluation of the MESMAC Project*, London: Health Education Authority.

ROONEY, M. and SCOTT, P. (1992) 'Working where the risks are: Health promotion interventions for gay men and other men who have sex with men in the second decade of the HIV epidemic', London: Health Education Authority (mimeo).

SCOTT, P. (1993) 'Beginning HIV-prevention work with gay and bisexual men', in EVANS, B., SANDBERG, S. and WATSON, S. (Eds) *Healthy Alliances in HIV Prevention*, London: Health Education Authority.

SHEFFIELD HEALTH AUTHORITY (1993) *Community Development and Health: The Way Forward in Sheffield*, Sheffield: Healthy Sheffield Support Team.

SIEGAL, K. and BAUMAN, L. (1986) 'Methodological issues in AIDS-related research, in FELDMAN, D. and JOHNSON, T. (Eds) *The Social Dimension of AIDS, Method and Theory*, London: Praeger.

SMITHIES, J. (1991) *Organisation and Community Development*, Unpublished Thesis, Sheffield Business School.

SMITHIES, J. and ADAMS, L. (1990) *Community Development and Health Education*, London: Health Education Authority.

WATNEY, S. (1987) 'People's perceptions of the risk of AIDS and the role of the mass media', *Health Education Journal*, **46**, 2, pp. 62–5.

WATNEY, S. (1988) 'Visual AIDS-advertising ignorance', in AGGLETON, P. and HOMANS, H. (Eds) *Social Aspects of AIDS*, Lewes: Falmer Press.

WATNEY, S. (1993) 'Emergent sexual identities and HIV/AIDS', in AGGLETON, P., DAVIES, P. and HART, G. (Eds.) *AIDS: Facing the Second Decade*, London: Falmer Press.

WEATHERBURN, P., HUNT, A., HICKSON, F.C.I. and DAVIES, P.M. (1992) *The Sexual Lifestyles of Gay and Bisexual Men in England and Wales*, London: Department of Health.

Katie Deverell, Alan Prout and Tom Doyle

WEEKS, J. (1989) 'AIDS, altruism, and the New Right', in CARTER, E. and WATNEY, S. (Eds) *Taking Liberties: AIDS and Cultural Politics*, London: Serpent's Tail.

WEEKS, J. (1990) 'The value of difference in RUTHERFORD, J. (Ed.) *Identity, Community, Culture, Difference*, London: Lawrence and Wishart.

WEBSTER, G. (1991) *Community Development and Health — A Collective Approach to Social Change*, Manchester, British Sociological Association Conference, Health and Safety.

Chapter 14

Selling Safer Sex: Male Masseurs and Escorts in the UK

Ford Hickson, Peter Weatherburn, Julian Hows and Peter Davies

Before the 1980s and the advent of HIV, most academic work on male prostitution treated it explicitly as a social problem. Descriptions were often prurient (especially Lloyd, 1979) and always condescending in their attitude to the population studied (Ginsburg, 1967; Caukins, 1974; Caukins and Coombs, 1976). This phenomenon is starkly illustrated in an article by Gandy and Deisher on the role of the physician in addressing this 'social problem', which begins:

> When [an earlier pilot study was] reported, the need for medical interest and leadership in the understanding and rehabilitation of these youths was expressed. Although the physician has little in his training or usual experience which would help him [sic] to recognize youths likely to engage in male prostitution or to counsel those living in this manner, he has the unique advantage in that he does not communicate the overwhelming disapproval these individuals assume from society in general.
>
> (Gandy and Deisher, 1970:1661)

A number of important points emerge from this brief extract: the easy assumption that medical practitioners should take the lead in defining and putting into effect the rehabilitation of these young men; the unquestioning acceptance of medical authority and legitimacy, despite the explicit inappropriateness of medical expertise and most obviously the lack of understanding masquerading as concern.

Two social changes in the 1970s–1980s rendered this approach old fashioned: first and emerging predominantly from within the feminist movement, the insistence on moving from a discourse of *prostitution*, concerned primarily with individual aetiology and the anatomy of a social problem, to one of *sex work* in which the economic and social constraints influencing those involved were given greater prominence (Barry, 1979). This shift in emphasis is profound and forms part of the larger challenge to hegemonic scientific attitudes posed by feminists, Black peoples, and others. Second and consequently, there has been a growing recognition of the diversity of male sex work (eg. Davies and Simpson, 1990; West and de Villiers, 1992; Marotta, Waldorf and Murphy, 1988; Estep, Waldorf and Marotta, 1992; Daniel and Parker, 1993).

Most notably, researchers began to describe forms of male sex work which do not accord the stereotypical notion of the indigent, impecunious, inexperienced young man, homeless and the victim of abuse who sells sex as a last bitter attempt to survive in a world which, when it is aware of his existence, is equally appalled by his predicament and insistent that he is to blame for it. These other sex workers depended on the existence of a large and complex gay community to create modes of work which allow a reasonable living to be made, and which also are carried out in some degree of comfort and with integrity (West and de Villiers, 1992).

Despite this, the majority of texts on male sex work and HIV concentrate on estimating the risk posed by this group of workers to the community at large — the 'general population' of traditional HIV epidemiology. Very recently, attention has started to be paid to the various cultural matrices within which male sex work occurs in a number of countries. This marks a welcome shift in perspective from the construction of sex workers as a threat to the health of the nation, to a concern with a group of workers whose chosen profession puts them, at least putatively and potentially, at enhanced risk of HIV infection. This chapter is an attempt to describe the HIV needs of a group of workers in the UK.

Male prostitution in the UK exists in a number of differing social forms. The most common of these include:

- Street-worker/client: younger workers, public venue negotiation, client controlled sex venue. Workers are commonly known as *rent-boys*.
- Freelancer/client: older workers, media advertised/telephone negotiated, negotiated sex venue. Workers are usually known as *masseurs* or *escorts*.
- Employee/agency/client: variable age of worker, mix of third person and direct negotiation via media, telephone, face-to-face, predetermined/ negotiated venue. Workers are usually known as *masseurs* or *escorts*.

While the operations of the different forms have been outlined (Davies and Simpson, 1990; West and de Villiers, 1992), most research has concentrated on those currently working as rent-boys. Sexual health outreach and advocacy work with people working as rent-boys is ongoing through a number of projects in Britain and is necessarily carried out within the context of a wide variety of other social and personal issues (housing, social skills, welfare benefits, for example). The social situation of men working as masseurs and escorts is thought to be considerably different to men working the streets, although how this influences sexual health advocacy work with this group is unexplored. How and why individuals move in and out of arrangements, what career paths exist, who act as clients and why, and differing sexual activities and risks associated with the roles are all largely unknown. We will be primarily concerned with freelancers, and the activities of people working as such. This is obviously related to the activities of clients, and to other roles in the overall picture of male prostitution.

Methods

London Lesbian and Gay Switchboard (LLGS) is a long established community-based information and support organization with high standing in the gay community. Project SIGMA is a seven year old research group investigating the socio-sexual responses of gay and bisexual men to HIV, and is again well known in the gay community. The work reported here took place between August 1992 and January 1993.

Using the opportunity of a mail-out of HIV education material by LLGS, a short questionnaire was distributed to men advertising in the gay press as masseurs and escorts. The questionnaire was designed: to provide baseline data on demographics, knowledge of HIV, sexual behaviour and sexual health; as a needs assessment indicating directions of possible future health promotion or advocacy work; and as an issue-raising exercise around sexual health, especially on the comparative risks between clients and non-paying partners.

Publications in which such advertisements are found were studied over a three week period, and again for one week after a lapse time of six weeks. Two hundred and eighty-six different personal advertisers' telephone numbers were located. Attempts were made by trained LLGS volunteers to contact all advertisers by telephone. Ninety-one per cent (260) were contacted and asked if they wanted to go on the LLGS list of 'personal service' providers, and if they would be willing to take part in an anonymous and confidential survey about masseur and escort work. Declining participation in the survey did not exclude entry on the database. Fifty-seven per cent (148) agreed to a database entry, and all but three of these agreed to take part in the survey. In addition, three respondents agreed to the survey but declined a listing. All were sent a covering letter, questionnaire and condom/lubricant pack. Fifty three questionnaires were returned by post, and fourteen questionnaires were completed by telephone.

Results

Of the 67 men returning the questionnaire, 79 per cent lived in London, the remainder coming from Newcastle, Manchester, Birmingham, Nottingham, Cardiff, Bristol and Lincoln. Two men returned the questionnaire in an unmarked envelope and their location could not be determined. The mean age of respondents was 28.6 (median 27; range 19–50). Half the men fell into the range 25–29. Most (88 per cent) were single, although 9 per cent have been in the past, and 3 per cent are currently, married. The majority (82 per cent) identified as gay, with the remainder identifying as bisexual. None claimed to be heterosexual or straight. Over half (58 per cent) lived alone, 21 per cent lived with a male sexual partner (one living with friends as well as his partner). The rest of the men lived with friends, except one man, who shared accommodation with other sex workers and their 'pimp', and one who lived with a female sexual partner and also shared with friends.

For just over half of the respondents, massage and sex work was their only work (54 per cent). Twenty-eight per cent also had a full time job, and fewer (18 per cent) did part-time work. Sixty-seven percent did not claim unemployment benefit. A quarter (24 per cent) said they did, and 9 per cent refused to answer. The most popular term nominated by the men to describe their work was masseur (67 per cent), closely followed by escort (46 per cent) and male prostitute (40 per cent). The terms model and rent boy were each nominated by only 10 per cent of men.[1] Four men preferred to use other descriptions of their work: entertainer/fantasy player, masseur offering extras, whore and counsellor.

Massage Work

Eighty two per cent said they offered a massage service. However, only half (53 per cent) of those had seen clients for only massage in the last week. Amongst those who had had massage-only clients in the previous week, the number of clients ranged from 1 to 30 (mean 5.7; median 4). Four respondents omitted the number of clients they had seen, one indicating he did not want his income worked out from his charges and the number of clients he had seen.

The mean cost of a massage (with no extras) was £39 (median £40; range £15–£65). Eight men declined to supply this data. The cost was on average £10 more if the masseur lived in London. The price of a massage was not associated with the age of the masseur.

Proportions Selling Sex and Age when Started

Of the 67 men answering the questionnaire, 61 (92 per cent) had sold sex at some point in their lives. Five men had not, and one refused to answer. Seventeen men made a distinction between the first time they were paid for sex, and the first time they sold sex. For those men the mean age of first being paid was 17.8 years (median 16; range 12–28). The mean time lag between being paid and selling for these men was 5.6 years (median 5; range 1–19), making their mean age at first selling the same as for the 72 per cent of men who did not make a distinction between getting paid and selling (that is, aged about 23 years).

The men had regularly been selling sex for a mean period of 3.6 years (median 3 years; range 5 months–12 years), although a third (33 per cent) had been selling for one year or less. Only one man who answered the questionnaire had sold sex in the past but did not do so currently (first paid aged 16, first sold aged 18, last sold aged 22, currently aged 24). This leaves 60 of the 67 returns currently selling sex.

Location of Work and Advertising

Virtually all of those currently selling sex, work from their own homes (97 per cent), as well as doing home or hotel visits (95 per cent). The most common conceptualization of their work was as 'a public service' (42 per cent). Thirty per cent think of it as a full time job, but slightly more (35 per cent) thought of it as a part time job. Very few men (5 per cent) thought of their sex work as a hobby. Although 22 per cent disliked doing the work but needed the money, more (30 per cent) liked the work in addition to getting paid, and 40 per cent said they did not mind the work. Not surprisingly, as this was how they were recruited, all the men advertised their services in the gay press, and 68 per cent also advertised in other ways. Around a quarter worked through agencies (28 per cent), or advertised in the non-gay (mainly local) press (20 per cent). Fewer men used telephone sex lines (8 per cent), newsagents' windows (7 per cent), and cards in public telephone booths (5 per cent).

Numbers of Clients

Ninety-five per cent had seen at least one client in the previous week. For those who had, the median number of clients was 6 (mean, 7.4; range 1–24). New clients had been seen by 95 per cent, and 83 per cent had seen a client they had seen before. For those who had seen that type of client in the preceding week, the median number of new clients was 3.5 (mean 4.4; range, 1–16), compared to a median of 2 (mean 3.3; range, 1–12) for regular clients.

Fewer men (47 per cent) had engaged in anal intercourse with a client in the preceding week. For those who had, the median number was 2 (mean 3.0; range, 1–11). Of those who had seen a client they had seen before, 40 per cent had anal intercourse with one or more of them, compared to 39 per cent of men who had seen new clients and engaged in anal intercourse with them. The proportions of regular and new clients with whom anal intercourse occurred was also very similar (20 per cent of regular clients compared to 18 per cent of new clients). Virtually all the men (97 per cent) said they had at least one regular client. The median number of regular clients was 10 (mean, 22; range, 0–500).

Sexual Practices with Clients

Table 14.1 presents the percentages of men who had engaged in each of twelve sexual acts. The first column gives the sexual act, the second column is the percentage of men who had ever engaged in that act with a client, and the third is the percentage who engaged in the last month (their current client repertoire). The rank order of lifetime repertoire and current repertoire are very similar, with only insertive anal intercourse with a condom and acting as an SM Bottom moving in the rank orderings. For convenience the sexual acts can be grouped into three: those which virtually all the men have done and are currently engaging in; those which most have done, but only some are currently doing; and those which few have done, and even fewer are currently engaged.

Masturbation of the client to orgasm and being fellated by a client are the staple of sexual activities for almost all male masseurs and escorts. These two acts are by far the most common amongst men that offer sexual services. The next group of acts are currently engaged in by between half and two-thirds of the men that currently sell sex, and have ever been engaged in by at least two thirds of all the men. These include both insertive and receptive anal intercourse using condoms, fellating the client, being masturbated to orgasm by the client, and acting as an SM top (the dominant partner in sadomasochistic sex).

The third group of uncommon acts comprise fellating the client to orgasm, insertive and receptive anal intercourse without condoms, and acting as an SM bottom (the submissive partner in sadomasochistic sex). Less than 10 per cent of men had done any of these acts in the last month, and none had engaged in receptive anal intercourse without a condom.

Table 14.1   Percentages engaging in sexual activities with clients, ever and in the last month

N = 60	Per cent ever	Per cent month
Masturbate him to orgasm	100	100
Be Fellated	98	95
Insertive A.I. condom	82	59
Fellated him	79	69
Be Masturbated to orgasm	78	69
Receptive A.I. condom	63	45
SM Top	62	45
Be Fellated to orgasm	52	25
Fellate him to orgasm	27	9
SM Bottom	18	7
IAI no condom	18	5
RAI no condom	11	0

AI = anal intercourse
IAI = insertive anal intercourse
RAI= receptive anal intercourse

Charges for Sexual Acts

Three men declined to specify any of their prices for sexual activities. Of the remaining 57, pricing systems varied. Forty per cent indicated a single flat charge which remained constant irrespective of the kind of sex that occurred. Flat charges ranged from £20 to £80 (median, £40; mean £46). A couple of men mentioned this charge being higher for 'call outs' than for the client coming to them. The remaining 60 per cent specified a sliding scale with different prices for different sexual acts. Most men (56 per cent of those with a sliding scale) used only two prices. For virtually all men with two prices, the lower price was charged for masturbation and fellatio, and the higher charge for anal intercourse and SM services. Nine men specified three prices, four specified four, and two specified five different prices.

Bearing in mind that not all acts were engaged in by all men, Table 14.2 gives the median, mean and range of prices for each of the sexual acts. All the median prices are between 40 and 55, and the general pattern that emerges in terms of increasing prices is: active and passive masturbation, being fellated, fellating a client, insertive anal intercourse, SM services, and receptive anal intercourse. The mean prices quoted for each act do not follow exactly the same pattern, as not all the men offered all the services, and the range of prices quoted was quite wide (cheapest masturbation £10, most expensive SM bottom service £1000).

Table 14.2   Average prices (£) for sexual acts, for those workers that will engage in them

N = 57	Mean	Median	Range
SM Bottom	124	50	20–1000
Receptive AI	64	40	40–150
Receptive. AI with Condom	62	55	15–200
Insertive AI	58	45	40–150
Insertive AI with Condom	55	50	20–125
SM Top	52	50	20–100
Be Fellated to Orgasm	49	45	20–100
Fellate him	47	50	10–100
Be fellated	45	45	10–100
Be masturbated	44	40	10–80
Masturbate him	43	40	20–80
Fellate him to orgasm	43	40	10–80

AI = Anal intercourse

As outlined in Table 14.1, the only universal act is masturbation of the client to orgasm, and it is also the cheapest. Amongst those who allowed themselves to be masturbated to orgasm by the client, a slightly higher mean charge is made, although the median is the same. Being fellated by the client is almost universally offered (95 per cent of men), although fewer are willing to fellate the client. Fellating the client is more expensive than being fellated, counting both the mean and median. Unusual effects are noticed if we look at fellatio to orgasm. Not all men who are willing to fellate or be fellated will allow the client to orgasm in their mouth, or come in theirs.

All but two of the 28 men who gave prices for being fellated charged the same whether they came in the clients mouth or not. Those two men specified £5 extra for coming in the client's mouth. Likewise, all but one of the 13 men giving prices for fellating the client charged the same whether the client came in their mouth or not (that one man charged an extra £30 when his clients orgasmed).

Most men (82 per cent) specified a price for insertive anal intercourse with a client with a condom, but fewer (63 per cent) were willing to be receptive, which was generally more expensive. Eight men specified a price for insertive anal intercourse without a condom, six of which specified the same price as with a condom, one indicating a lower price without a condom, and one specifying a much higher price. Five did for receptive anal intercourse without a condom. These five were all included in the eight who specified a price for anal intercourse without a condom.

Table 14.3 Male non-paying sexual partners in the preceding month: percentages having them and their average numbers

N = 60	Per cent	Median	Mean	Range
Regular partners	63	1.5	2.1	1–10
Casual partners	70	4	5.7	1–20
AI with Regular	42	1	2.1	1–10
AI with Casual	47	2.5	3.6	1–15

AI = anal intercourse

Non-paying Sexual Partners

Sixty per cent currently had at least one regular male sexual partner who was not a client. A further 7 per cent currently had both regular male and regular female non-paying partners. Of those with a regular partner, 68 per cent said their partners knew about their sex work, and a further 23 per cent said some partners did and some did not. Only 9 per cent said none of their regular partners know about their sex work.

Ninety-four per cent had had sex with male non-paying partners in the preceding month (for those who had, the median number of partners was 4; mean, 5.8; range, 1–23), and 70 per cent had male non-paying penetrative partners (median, 2; mean, 3.8; range, 1–20). Table 14.3 gives the numbers of male non-paying sexual partners for the preceding month. As with clients, more men had seen casual partners than had seen regular partners, and those who had casual partners had more of them. Only 3 had sex with a female non-paying partner, all of whom had engaged in vaginal intercourse with that partner.

Sexual Health

The vast majority (88 per cent) had attended an STD or GUM clinic at some time in the past. Of those who had, 84 per cent had attended at least once in the last year. Table 14.4 gives percentages of men ever having had a number of sexually transmitted infections (STDs). The most common STDs were gonorrhoea and NSU, with 68 per cent having had a past infection with one or both of these. Twenty-eight per cent report never having had any of these infections

Almost half the men (49 per cent) had received hepatitis B vaccinations, with a further 20 per cent knowing they were naturally immune. Eighty-four per cent of respondents had had an HIV antibody test at some point in the past,

Table 14.4 Percentage of men reporting ever having had sexually transmitted infections

Infections	Per cent ever
Gonorrhoea	52
NSU	50
Genital Warts	25
Hepatitis	13
Herpes	12
Syphilis	7

NSU = non-specific urethritis

higher than the current estimate for gay men in general. Of those that had tested, half (51 per cent) said they went for HIV antibody tests regularly.

Safer Sex and Condom Use

When asked how seriously they took safer sex with both clients and non-paying sexual partners, men indicated that they took it more seriously with clients. On a four-point scale, 83 per cent said they took safer sex 'very seriously' with clients, but only 59 per cent said they take it 'very seriously' with non-paying partners. Very few said they take safer sex 'not very seriously' with either clients or other partners, and none said they take it 'not at all seriously'.

Use of condoms for anal intercourse in the last year are given in Table 14.5. The incidence of receptive anal intercourse is lower than insertive for all partner types, but with larger differences with clients. Amongst clients, condom use for both insertive and receptive is more common with casual clients than with regular clients, but condom use is almost universal for anal intercourse with clients. Four of the 60 men had had anal intercourse with a client without a condom in the preceding year.

Summary and discussion

A number of important points emerge from these data. This group of men who sell sex advertising as masseurs and escorts are predominantly gay-identified, in their late 20s, housed, and the majority either do not mind or enjoy their sex work. That the major motivation for their work is not economic necessity is reflected in the finding that for only a quarter is massage and sex work their only income. Another quarter also claim state benefits, while half also have other jobs. Most men started selling sex in their early twenties, and had not been paid for sex before they sold it. This suggests their sex work is not opportunistic, and that there is not a rent-boy/masseur career path. About half consider themselves to be providing a public service. All the above suggest most masseurs and escorts are young men making positive premeditated decisions to sell sex, in the context of other financial alternatives. Their social and economic situation is therefore very different from the stereotypical, indigent rent-boys.

These masseurs and escorts are a group of gay and bisexual men who are very sexually active, with both paying and non-paying partners. The average masseur will have seen three new clients, and two (of his 10) regular clients in the last week, and he will have engaged in anal intercourse with at most one of these. The bulk of sex work consists of masturbating the client and being fellated by him. The majority of masseurs offer anal intercourse (more offer insertive than receptive) but few offer anal intercourse without condoms, and fewer have done it in the past month (5 per cent insertive, none receptive). This discrepancy in condom use by mode of anal intercourse may reflect men's greater willingness to engage in unprotected insertive anal intercourse than receptive, and would be in line with the generally held view that acquiring HIV is more difficult as the insertive rather than the receptive partner.

The proportion of men with regular non-paying partners (lovers and boyfriends) is comparable with gay men generally (Davies *et al.*, 1993). However, more men had casual non-paying partners. In addition to clients, the average masseur will have sex with 4 5 non-paying partners in a month, one or two of whom will be a regular partner. This is considerably higher than gay men in general, but this is a group of younger, non-monogamous men, who are likely to have more partners irrespective of sex work. What is different amongst these men from the general population of gay men, is that their casual penetrative partners outnumber their regular ones. Slightly more men had a casual penetrative sexual partner (PSP) in the preceding month, than had had a regular one. Also, amongst those with PSPs, casual ones account for more than twice the number of regulars. The high number of sexual partners and PSPs should give concern for the sexual health of these men. However, it is important not to immediately categorize them as at high risk for all infections, especially HIV. While their high rate of partner change may bring them into contact with sexual partners with infectious agents, their ability to cope with this likelihood should not be underestimated.

Their knowledge of HIV and safer sex is high, there is a high rate of GUM clinic attendance, and the proportion having taken HIV antibody tests is very high. This is a group of men knowledgable about sexual health: after all, it is their business. As with research on other groups of male sex workers, masseurs took safer sex with clients more seriously than with non-paying partners. This is reflected in condom use being higher with clients. Only 7 per cent had had anal intercourse with a client without a condom in the last year, whereas 23 per cent had anal intercourse with a non-paying partner without a condom (18 per cent had done so with a casual non-paying partner). However, condom use is higher

Table 14.5 Condom use with clients and non-paying partners for IAI and RAI in the preceeding year

N = 60	Per cent AI	Percent Condom always	Percent Condom sometimes	Percent Condom never
IAI Regular Client	67	93	7	0
RAI Regular Client	50	93	7	0
IAI Casual Client	77	96	4	0
RAI Casual Client	55	94	6	0
IAI Regular Non-paying	70	76	22	2
RAI Regular Non-paying	62	78	19	3
IAI Casual Non-paying	78	77	23	0
RAI Casual Non-paying	72	79	21	0

IAI = Insertive anal intercourse
RAI = Receptive anal intercourse

with non-paying male partners amongst these men than it is amongst gay men generally.

Ongoing sexual health advocacy work with this group is desirable given their large number of sexual partners, and while high clinic attendance and preventative measures such as hepatitis B vaccination uptake are not universal. Given the above, masseurs and escorts are best regarded as expert safer sex practitioners, and potential peer and client educators. This is a group of gay men, whose average working time is a few years, starting in their early twenties, coming from and remaining part of the gay scene. Consequently, this may be best achieved by ongoing safer sex promotion amongst gay men.

An unexplored safer sex educational technique could also be the encouragement of these men as educators to their clients. While little is known about the clients of these men, we may speculate that they include men who are either closeted, non-gay identified, or have little access to the gay scene, and its wealth of safer sex information and peer norms.

Note

1   Percentages do not total to 100, as some men nominated more than one term.

Acknowledgements

This work was begun with a very small grant from the Health Education Authority and subsequently funded by South East London Health Promotion

Service (now Health First: Health Promotion in Lambeth, Lewisham, and Southwark) and North East Thames Regional Health Authority. The views and opinions expressed herein are those of the authors only.

References

BARRY, K., (1979) *Female Sexual Slavery*, New York: Avon.

CAUKINS, N.R. (1974) 'Male prostitution: a psychosocial view of behaviour', *American Journal of Orthopsychiatry*, **44**, pp. 782–5.

CAUKINS, S.E. and COOMBS, N.R. (1976) 'The psychodynamics of male prostitution', *The American Journal of Psychotherapy*, **30**, pp. 782–9.

DANIEL, H. and PARKER, R. (1993) *Sexuality, Politics and AIDS in Brazil*, London: Falmer Press.

DAVIES, P.M. and SIMPSON, P. (1990) 'On Male Homosexual Prostitution and HIV', in AGGLETON, P., DAVIES, P.M. and HART, G. (Eds) *AIDS: Individual, Cultural and Policy Dimensions*, London: Falmer Press.

DAVIES, P.M., HICKSON, F.C.I., WEATHERBURN, P. and HUNT, A.J. (1993) *Sex, Gay Men and AIDS*, London: Falmer Press.

ESTEP, R., WALDORF, D., and MAROTTA, T. (1992) 'Sexual behaviour of male prostitutes', in HUBER, J. and SCHNEIDER, B.E. (Eds) *The Social Context of AIDS*, London: Sage.

GANDY, P. and DEISHER, R. (1970) 'Young male prostitutes: The physicians role in social rehabilitation', *Journal of the American Medical Association*, **212**, 10, pp. 1661–6.

GINSBURG, K.N. (1967) 'The "meat-rack": a study of the male homosexual prostitute', *American Journal of Psychotherapy*, **21**, pp. 170–85.

LLOYD, R. (1979) *Playland: A Study of Human Exploitation*, London: Quartet.

MAROTTA, T., WALDORF, D., MURPHY, S. (1988) 'Males doing sex-work in the San Francisco Bay area: A typology and description', unpublished paper, San Francisco, CA: Institute for scientific analysis.

WEST, D.J. and DE VILLIERS, B. (1992) *Male Prostitution*, London: Duckworth.

Contributors

Peter Aggleton is Reader in Education at Goldsmiths' College, University of London, and co-director of the Health and Education Research Unit at the Institute of Education, University of London. He has worked extensively in HIV/AIDS health promotion. His publications include *Deviance* (Tavistock, 1987); *Health* (Routledge, 1990); *AIDS: Responses, Interventions and Care* (Ed. with Graham Hart and Peter Davies, Falmer, 1991); *AIDS: Rights, Risk and Reason* (Ed. with Peter Davies and Graham Hart, Falmer, 1992); and *AIDS: Facing the Second Decade* (Ed. with Peter Davies and Graham Hart, Falmer, 1993).

Augustine Ankomah is a lecturer in Population Studies at the Institute of Population Studies, University of Exeter. His current research interests include sexual health, particularly the sexual behaviour of young women in West Africa and its implications for HIV transmission and prevention. He is currently undertaking an experimental community-based HIV intervention project in south west Nigeria funded by the AIDSCAP division of Family Health International.

Michael Bartos is a higher degree student at La Trobe University, Melbourne, researching the intersection of the government of sexuality and of public health, as it has been reorganized by HIV/AIDS. His research is supported by a scholarship from the Commonwealth AIDS Research Grants Committee. He is also President of the Victorian AIDS Council/Gay Men's Health Centre and a committee member of the Australian Federation of AIDS Organisations.

Peter Davies is Director of Research in the School of Health Studies at the University of Portsmouth. He is a Principal Investigator of Project SIGMA

(Socio-sexual Investigations of Gay Men and AIDS) and author of *Key Texts in Multidimensional Scaling* (Heinemann, 1982); *Images of Social Stratification* (Sage, 1985); and co-author (with Ford Hickson, Peter Weatherburn and Andrew Hunt) of *Sex, Gay Men and AIDS* (Falmer, 1993). He is editor (with Peter Aggleton and Graham Hart) of *AIDS: Social Representations, Social Practices* (Falmer, 1989); *AIDS: Individual, Cultural and Policy Dimensions* (Falmer, 1990); *AIDS: Responses, Interventions and Care* (Falmer, 1991); *AIDS: Risk, Rights and Reason* (Falmer, 1992); and *AIDS: Facing the Second Decade* (Falmer, 1993).

Katie Deverell is currently undertaking an evaluation of the Terrence Higgins Trust's Roadshow project. She is also a research student in the Department of Sociology and Social Anthropology at Keele University where she is studying the construction of sexual boundaries at work. Recent publications include a paper in *Practising Anthropology*, and (with Alan Prout) *MESMAC Working with Diversity — Building Communities, An Evaluation of a Community Development Approach to HIV Prevention for Men who have Sex with Men* (HEA, forthcoming).

Tom Doyle manages the Leeds MESMAC Project and is co-ordinator of Yorkshire MESMAC, one of England's largest gay men's health projects. Recent publications include (with Katie Deverell) *MESMAC Leeds: An Evaluation of the Establishment of a Lesbian and Gay Theatre Group, MESMAC Evaluation Working Paper No. 6* (Keele University, 1992).

Nicholas Ford is a lecturer in Population Studies at the Institute of Population Studies, University of Exeter. He undertakes research into sexual and fertility-regulating behaviour, HIV risk-reduction strategies and prevention. His primary areas of overseas research interest are South East Asia and Ghana. He is consultant on sexual behaviour research to the South Western Regional Health Authority. He has contributed articles to journals including the *Journal of Epidemiology and Community Medicine, Social Science and Medicine* and the *British Journal of Family Planning*.

David Goss is Reader in Organizational Behaviour and co-Director of the Centre for AIDS and Employment Research, University of Portsmouth Business School. He has published numerous articles on HIV/AIDS and employment, and is currently writing a book on this subject with Derek Adam-Smith. He has also published books on small firm employment relations and human resource management.

Gill Green is a researcher at the MRC Medical Sociology Unit, University of Glasgow. She is working on a follow-up study of a sample of men and women with HIV in Scotland which focuses on the psychosocial impact of an

HIV-positive diagnosis and styles of stigma management. She is interested in cross-cultural comparisons and is currently trying to develop links with other researchers in Europe.

Ford Hickson is a research fellow with Project SIGMA (Socio-sexual Investigations of Gay Men and AIDS) based in South London and affiliated to the University of Essex. His main research areas are HIV and patterns of gay male relationships, and sexual assault amongst men. He is the instigator and compiler of *The Directory of Lesbian and Gay Studies in the UK*, and co-author (with Peter Davies, Peter Weatherburn and Andrew Hunt) of *Sex, Gay Men and AIDS* (Falmer, 1993).

Julian V. Hows has been a gay activist for more than 20 years. He has been involved with London Lesbian and Gay Switchboard (LLGS) for 13 years, and is currently its vice-chair. At present he is engaged in research and sexual health outreach with non-street working male sex workers in London, as part of the joint Project SIGMA and LLGS initiative, Working with London's Male Masseurs and Escorts'. In another life he is Sister Divine Revelation OPI (Order of Perpetual Indulgence).

Charles Nzioka is a doctoral student in the Department of Sociology at Goldsmiths' College, University of London, and a lecturer in sociology at the University of Nairobi, Kenya.

Alan Prout is a senior lecturer in the Department of Sociology and Social Anthropology at Keele University, and Course Director for the Centre for Medical Social Anthropology. Recent publications include a chapter in *Does it Work? Perspectives on the Evaluation of HIV/AIDS Health Promotion*, (P. Aggleton *et al.*, Eds, HEA, 1992) and (with Katie Deverell) in *MESMAC Working with Diversity — Building Communities, An Evaluation of a Community Development Approach to HIV Prevention for Men who have Sex with Men* (HEA, forthcoming).

Tim Rhodes is a research fellow at the Centre for Research on Drugs and Health Behaviour, Charing Cross and Westminster Medical School. He is currently conducting qualitative research on risk, sexual health and sexual negotiation among illicit drug users and their sexual partners. Recent publications include *HIV Prevention and Illicit Drug Use: Developments in Research and Health Promotion Strategy* (London, Health Education Authority, 1994). He is co-editor (with Richard Hartnoll) of *HIV Prevention in the Community: Perspectives on Individual, Community and Political Action* (Routledge, in press).

Neil Small is a senior research fellow at York University's Social Policy Research Unit. He is the author of *Politics and Planning in the National Health Service* (Open University Press, 1989); *AIDS: The Challenge. Understanding, Education and Care* (Avebury, 1993). He is currently involved in research on the interface of health and social care.

Derek Adam-Smith is a senior lecturer in Human Resource Management and Co-Director of the Centre for AIDS and Employment Research, University of Portsmouth Business School. He has published a number of papers on HIV/AIDS and the workplace, and is co-author (with David Goss) of a forthcoming book on this subject.

Austin Taylor-Laybourn is a research officer in the Health and Education Research Unit at the Institute of Education, University of London. He is currently working on an ESRC funded project concerning voluntary sector responses to HIV and AIDS, and has recently completed a local HIV/AIDS health promotion needs assessment research project for men who have sex with men commissioned by Camberwell Health Authority.

Peter Weatherburn is a social psychologist and a senior research officer with Project SIGMA based in South London. He has worked extensively in the field of HIV and sexual health research, recently concentrating on localized HIV policy research. He is co-author (with Peter Davies, Ford Hickson and Andrew Hunt) of *Sex, Gay Men and AIDS* (Falmer, 1993).

Jeffrey Weeks is Professor of Social Relations and Director of the Centre for Social and Economic Research at the University of the West of England, Bristol. He is the author of numerous articles and books on various aspects of the social regulation of sexuality. These include *Coming Out* (Quartet, 1977 and 1990); *Sex, Politics and society* (Longman, 1981 and 1989); *Sexuality and its Discontents* (Routledge and Kegan Paul, 1985); *Sexuality* (Tavistock, 1986); *Between the Acts: Lives of Homosexual Men 1985–1967* (with Kevin Porter, Routledge, 1991); and *Against Nature: Essays on History, Sexuality and Identity* (Rivers Oram Press, 1991). He is currently working on a book on sexual values, and is co-director (with Peter Aggleton) of an ESRC funded project examining voluntary sector responses to HIV/AIDS.

Daniel Wight is a researcher at the MRC Medical Sociology Unit at the University of Glasgow. His research interests include working class culture, consumption, risk, sexuality, and HIV in Uganda. He is currently working on sexual health interventions. He is author of *Workers not Wasters: Masculine Respectability, Consumption and Unemployment in Scotland* (Edinburgh University Press, 1993); and co-author (with P. McMichael and B. Lynch) of *Building Bridges into Work* (Longman, 1990).

Carla Willig is a lecturer in psychology at Middlesex University. She has recently completed her doctoral thesis entitled *AIDS: A Study of the Social Construction of Knowledge*. Her research and teaching interests include discourse analytic work in psychology. She is currently conducting research into the meanings and practices of trust in romantic relationships.

Index